Don't Fall!
I'm Falling !

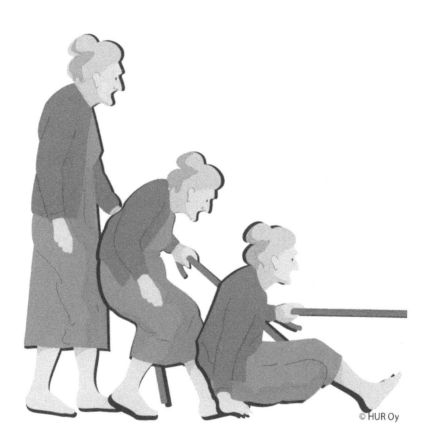

© HUR Oy

Falling, but I'm getting up
Chronicle of Older
Adults/Seniors Falls.

MC Griffin Campbell, M.Div., MA

Don't Fall!
I'm Falling but, I'm getting up!

To all Older Adults 60 years and above
Purpose: To Give a detailed account of the dangers of Falls to help save the lives of "Older Adults."
Helping save the lives of "Older Adults" must start with the power of knowing God and His word.
Awareness, the knowing and the resurrection power of the Holy Spirit raises us up and causes us to stand up again when we fall down is to bring in the God-Factor-our major defense.

Don't Fall!
I'm Falling but, I'm getting up!

Table of Contents

Don't Fall!
I'm Falling but, I'm getting up!

Don't Fall!
I'm Falling but, I'm getting up!

Introduction

A Bible Story of a young man falling 3 stories. As a result, he was declared "all right" by Paul. Resurrection
[8] The upstairs room where we met was lighted with many flickering lamps; [9] and as Paul spoke on and on, a young man named Eutychus, sitting on the windowsill, went fast asleep and fell three stories to his death below. [10-12] Paul went down and took him into his arms. "Don't worry," he said, "he's all right!" And he was! What a wave of awesome joy swept through the crowd!
Acts20:8-12.

Don't Fall!
I'm Falling but, I'm getting up!

This book has a 3-fold purpose:
To bring Awareness on the seriousness of Senior Falls.
To help educate Seniors on Falling and the consequences.
To help prevent Seniors from Falling Injuries.
Our goal is to end Older Adults' falls, injury and death related serious injuries, disability and even deaths.

Falls are the leading cause of fatal and non-fatal injuries for older Americans. Falls threaten Seniors' safety and independence and generate enormous economic and personal costs.

For these reasons, we must be committed to gaining Wisdom, Understanding and Knowledge of difficult issues of Older Adults' Falls;
First and foremost, bringing in the God Factor-a must- Seeking His word and His presence in all things:
The Power of Awareness must be kept front and center
Education in "Older Adult" Falls
Training the community and "Older Adults" Safety and well-being

6

Don't Fall!
I'm Falling but, I'm getting up!

Prevention of Falls
Falls leading to serious injuries, disability and even Deaths
Statistical data, Solutions and safety tips that can save lives.

Quotes
Older Adults & Falls

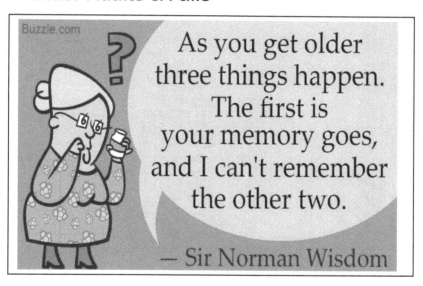

As you get older three things happen. The first is your memory goes, and I can't remember the other two.

— Sir Norman Wisdom

Don't Fall!
I'm Falling but, I'm getting up!

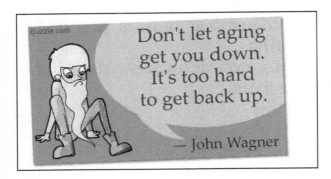

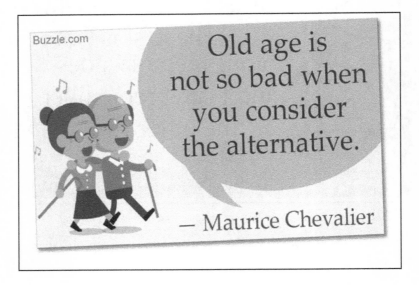

"

Don't Fall!
I'm Falling but, I'm getting up!

To make an elderly person happy is the noblest act a young person can ever do!"
— Mehmet Murat ilda
"It always a blessing to learn the wisdom from elderly people."
— Lailah Gifty Akita

"Blessed are you when you enjoyed the company of elderly people. They are always ready to share their rich experience and wisdom with young people."
— Lailah Gifty Akita

"It always a blessing to learn the wisdom from elderly people."
— Lailah Gifty Akita

"Failing is not an option and falling either. But to get up after a fall otherwise is what's in a mind of a winner!"
— Ana Claudia Antunes,

"To fall down is to face the weakness of my humanity, test the mettle of my character, and push the limits of my strength. Therefore, falling down will tell me who I am far more clearly than most

Don't Fall!
I'm Falling but, I'm getting up!

things I might learn when I'm standing
up."
— Craig D. Lounsbrough

"I much prefer not to fall, unless of course
I am falling into the hands of God."
— Craig D. Lounsbrough

"Sometimes it takes a good fall to really
know where you stand"
— Hayley Williams

"You can't become a decent horseman
until you fall off and get up again, a good
number of times.
There's life in a nutshell."
— Bear Grylls, <u>Mud, Sweat and Tears</u>

"And falling's just another way to fly."
— Emilie Autumn
"Lessons are learned through making
mistakes, falling and rising."
— Sunday Adelaja

"Strength is about pulling yourself
together, even after you've been
shattered into a thousand pieces. Falling
is merely the first movement we take

Don't Fall!
I'm Falling but, I'm getting up!

before rising" — Rehan Khan, A Tudor
Turk
"Falling isn't so bad, you know. It's only
the landing that hurts."
— Terry Pratchett, The Color of Magic

Jeannette Walls
People who fall the hardest, bounce back
the highest." – Nishan Panwar.
"Just because we fell one time doesn't
mean we can't get up and let our light
shine."
"When real people fall down in life, they
get right back up and keep walking."
"It's hard to beat a person that never
gives up."

God's word on Falling Down.

Proverbs 24:16 ESV /
For the righteous falls seven times and
rises again, but the wicked stumble in
times of calamity.
Luke 17:16 ESV / 14
And he fell on his face at Jesus' feet,
giving him thanks. Now he was a
Samaritan.

Don't Fall!
I'm Falling but, I'm getting up!

<u>Joshua 5:14</u> ESV / 9
And he said, "No; but I am the commander of the army of the LORD. Now I have come." And Joshua fell on his face to the earth and worshiped and said to him, "What does my lord say to his servant?"
<u>Acts 9:4-6</u> ESV / 7
And falling to the ground he heard a voice saying to him, "Saul, Saul, why are you persecuting me?" And he said, "Who are you, Lord?" And he said, "I am Jesus, whom you are persecuting. But rise and enter the city, and you will be told what you are to do."
<u>Matthew 26:39</u> ESV / 7
And going a little farther he fell on his face and prayed, saying, "My Father, if it be possible, let this cup pass from me; nevertheless, not as I will, but as you will."
<u>Matthew 17:6</u> ESV / 7
When the disciples heard this, they fell on their faces and were terrified.

<u>2 Chronicles 20:18</u> ESV / 6
Then Jehoshaphat bowed his head with his face to the ground, and all Judah and the inhabitants of Jerusalem fell down before the LORD, worshiping the LORD.
<u>Numbers 20:6</u>

Don't Fall!
I'm Falling but, I'm getting up!

Then Moses and Aaron went from the presence of the assembly to the entrance of the tent of meeting and fell on their faces. And the glory of the LORD appeared to them,
Numbers 16:4 ESV / 6
When Moses heard it, he fell on his face,
Mark 14:35 ESV / 5
And going a little farther, he fell on the ground and prayed that, if it were possible, the hour might pass from him.
Matthew 7:7 ESV / 5
"Ask, and it will be given to you; seek, and you will find; knock, and it will be opened to you.
Ezekiel 1:28 ESV / 5
Like the appearance of the bow that is in the cloud on the day of rain, so was the appearance of the brightness all around. Such was the appearance of the likeness of the glory of the LORD. And when I saw it, I fell on my face, and I heard the voice of one speaking.

Leviticus 9:24 ESV /
And fire came out from before the LORD and consumed the burnt offering and the pieces of fat on the altar, and

Don't Fall!
I'm Falling but, I'm getting up!

when all the people saw it, they shouted
and fell on their faces.

Genesis 17:17 ESV

Then Abraham fell on his face and
laughed and said to himself, "Shall a child
be born to a man who is a hundred years
old? Shall Sarah, who is ninety years old,
bear a child?"

John 18:6 "when Jesus said to them, "I am
he," they drew back and fell to the ground

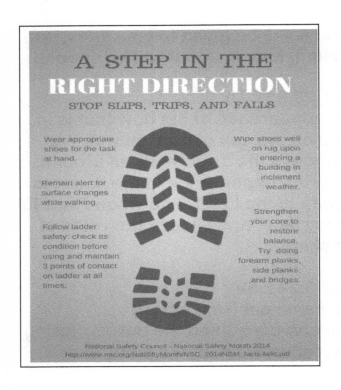

Don't Fall!
I'm Falling but, I'm getting up!

<u>Resurrection in Old Age Falls</u>
The Lord will help us stand up in our Falls

<u>Resurrection refers to standing up again</u>
<u>Resurrection</u>

Resurrection power is in God's word. He teaches us to stand again.

comeback, snapback, return to health, getting better, gaining strength, getting well, on the mend, to stand again; the <u>act</u> or <u>fact</u> of <u>bringing</u> someone back to <u>life</u>, or <u>bringing</u> something back into use or <u>existence</u>: the <u>act</u> of <u>bringing</u> something that had <u>disappeared</u> or <u>ended</u> back into use or <u>existence</u>

1. <u>Proverbs</u> 24:16 for though a righteous man falls seven times, he will rise again, but the wicked stumble into calamity.

2. Psalm 37:23-24 The LORD directs the steps of the godly. He delights in every detail of their lives. Though they stumble, they will never fall, for the LORD holds them by the hand.

Don't Fall!
I'm Falling but, I'm getting up!

3. Psalm 145:14-16 The LORD helps the fallen and lifts those bent beneath their loads. The eyes of all look to you in hope; you

Psalm 20:8 Those nations will fall down and collapse, but we will rise up and stand firm.

7. Psalm 63:7-8 for you have been my help, and in the shadow of your wings I will sing for joy. My soul clings to you; your right hand upholds me.

8. 2 Samuel 22:37 You have made a wide path for my feet to keep them from slipping.

9. Isaiah 41:13 For I the LORD thy God will hold thy right hand, saying unto thee, Fear not; I will help thee.

10. Psalm 37:17 for the power of the wicked will be broken, but the LORD upholds the righteous.

Live by God's Word and you will not stumble.

Don't Fall!
I'm Falling but, I'm getting up!

11. Proverbs 3:22-23 My son, do not lose sight of these— keep sound wisdom and discretion, then you will walk on your way securely, and your foot will not stumble.

12. Psalm 119:165 Those who love your instructions have great peace and do not stumble.

13. Proverbs 4:11-13 I will teach you wisdom's ways and lead you in straight paths. When you walk, you won't be held back; when you run, you won't stumble. Take hold of my instructions; don't let them go. Guard them, for they are the key to life.

What is God saying about Older Adults-

Proverbs 16:31 Gray hair is a crown of splendor; it is attained in the way of righteousness.

Isaiah 46:4 Even to your old age and gray hairs I am he, I am he who will sustain you. I have made you and I will carry you; I will sustain you and I will rescue you.

Job 12:12 Is not wisdom found among the aged? Does not long-life bring understanding?

Don't Fall!
I'm Falling but, I'm getting up!

Deuteronomy 32:7. Remember the days of old; consider the generations long past. Ask your father and he will tell you, your elders, and they will explain to you
1 Timothy 5:17 The elders who direct the affairs of the church well are worthy of double honor, especially those whose work is preaching and teaching.
Psalm 71:18 Even when I am old and gray, do not forsake me, my God, till I declare your power to the next generation, your mighty acts to all who are to come.
II Timothy 4:7-8 I have fought the good fight, I have finished the race, I have kept the faith. Now there is in store for me the crown of righteousness, which the Lord, the righteous Judge, will award to me on that day—and not only to me, but also to all who have longed for his appearing. give them their food as they need it. When you open your hand, you satisfy the hunger and thirst of every living thing.

14. Psalm 119:45 I will walk about in freedom, for I have sought out your precepts.
15. Jeremiah 8:4 "Say to them, 'This is what the LORD says: "'When people fall

Don't Fall!
I'm Falling but, I'm getting up!

down, do they not get up? When someone turns away, do they not return?

16. 2 Corinthians 4:8-10 We are pressured in every way but not crushed; we are perplexed but <u>not in despair</u>, we are persecuted but not abandoned; we are struck down but not destroyed. We always carry the death of Jesus in our body, so that the life of Jesus may also be revealed in our body.

17. Ecclesiastes 4:9-12 Two people are better than one because together they have a <u>good reward for their hard work</u>. 10 If one falls, the other can help his friend get up. But how tragic it is for the one who is all alone when he falls. There is no one to help him get up. Again, if two people lie down together, they can keep warm, but how can one person keep warm? Though one person may be overpowered by another, two people can resist one opponent. A triple-braided rope is not easily broken.

18. Romans 3:23 for all have sinned and fall short of the glory of God.

Don't Fall!
I'm Falling but, I'm getting up!

19. 1 Corinthians 10:13 No temptation has overtaken you that is unusual for human beings. But God is faithful, and he will not allow you to be tempted beyond your strength. Instead, along with the temptation he will also provide a way out, so that you may be able to endure it

Do not rejoice when your enemy falls.
20. Proverbs 24:17 Don't gloat when your enemy falls, and don't let your heart rejoice when he stumbles.

21. Micah 7:8 Do not gloat over me, my enemies! For though I fall, I will rise again. Though I sit in darkness, the LORD will be my light.
https://biblereasons.com/falling/https://www.patheos.com/blogs/christiancrier/2015/06/24/top-7-bible-verses-about-old-age-or-the-elderly/

I Thess. 4:14 For we believe that Jesus died and rose again, and so we believe that God will bring with Jesus those who have fallen asleep in him
Matt. 28: 5-6 The angel said to the women, "Do not be afraid, for I know that you are looking for Jesus, who was crucified. He

Don't Fall!
I'm Falling but, I'm getting up!

is not here; he has risen, just as he said. Come and see the place where he lay." Hebrews 13: 20-21 Now may the God of peace, who through the blood of the eternal covenant brought back from the dead our Lord Jesus, that great Shepherd of the sheep, equip you with everything good for doing his will, and may he work in us what is pleasing to him, through Jesus Christ, to whom be glory for ever and ever. Amen.
Acts 26:22 But God has helped me to this very day; so, I stand here and testify to small and great alike. I am saying nothing beyond what the prophets and Moses said would happen— that the Messiah would suffer and, as the first to rise from the dead, would bring the message of light to his own people and to the Gentiles.
Rev. 20:12 And I saw the dead, great and small, standing before the throne, and books were opened. Another book was opened, which is the book of life. The dead were judged according to what they had done as recorded in the books. The sea gave up the dead that were in it, and death and Hades gave up the dead that were in them, and each person was judged according to what they had done.

Don't Fall!
I'm Falling but, I'm getting up!

Author Notes.

Older Adults Falls can sometimes result to serious injuries.

Each Fall is different. Some inside the home-some outside-walking, running, playing baseball with grandchildren, playing in the park, missing a step or two-Falls can happen.

All of these are minors, however there are other falls that are serious-can be serious that can lead to mobility issues and sometimes even deaths.

I believe Awareness is our best defense; education and prevention working together can bring the Victory.
Now I like to share our story of falls:

Gene's Story: The most painful one (there were others)
While walking with his hands full with clothes coming from the dry cleaners going to the car in the parking lot; he stumbled or tripped over cement parking lot and fell onto sidewalk bruising his chin.

Don't Fall!
I'm Falling but, I'm getting up!

According to Gene, he felled down the stairs on the job; several falls inside the home and a few other outside, there were (1) fall in the workplace, a few others inside the home. No broken bones or serious injuries, all were minors.

My Story: My Last Fall
On May 11, 2018, 11:00 am, I was walking in the lobby of Insurance company-on my way to the elevator- to go up on the 5th floor to my doctor's office.
As I passed the long reception counter, there were people scattered around the area talking to each other. As I preceded to turn the corner to get to the elevator, I slipped up on something-not sure what, but as I felled forward -My hands were stretched out and landed on the checked tile floor. I hit the floor so hard I saw dust fly up from the floor below. There seemed to be a bouncing effect as I landed on my left side. There was no major pain after the fall-only little stingy pain left knee area. As a result, a pinched nerve. As a result, a pinched nerve which was diagnosed as spinal stenosis.Be in the Know For your Information: What is Spinal

Don't Fall!
I'm Falling but, I'm getting up!

Stenosis. There is a lot of pain-here are some symptoms I am experiencing even today.

Don't Fall!
I'm Falling but, I'm getting up!

Ten Symptoms of Spinal Stenosis.

Spinal stenosis refers to a narrowing of the spinal canal leading to compression of the spinal nerve roots or the spinal cord. There are two types of stenosis: lumbar and cervical. In both cases, affected individuals experience symptoms relating to the nerves of the spinal cord. Because most nerves travel through the spinal column, <u>symptoms</u> can be wide-ranging and affect the entire body.

1. Pain While Walking
One of the most common symptoms of spinal stenosis is a <u>pain</u> in the leg while walking or pseudo claudication.
Upright <u>exercise</u> and prolonged standing can worsen this symptom, which usually progresses over time and eases as soon as the person sits down. This pain often leads to diminished activity. Physical therapy and specific changes in posture may help reduce this symptom.

2. Tingling Sensations

Don't Fall!
I'm Falling but, I'm getting up!

Another frequent <u>symptom</u> of spinal stenosis is a tingling sensation in the legs or arms, or throughout the entire body. Most people compare the feeling to pins and needles. This symptom develops due to reduced blood flow, which causes areas to "fall asleep." Stretching the affected body part gently can help alleviate the sensation, though sudden movements can provoke it or make it worse.

3. Pain in the Neck 6. Waves of Pain
The type of <u>pain</u> spinal stenosis causes varies from person to person. Many report pains that comes in intense and temporary waves that typically last a few hours, though some flare-ups can last for days. A physician may recommend <u>applying</u> a cold pack to the affected area and restricting movement as much as possible when a person with spinal stenosis is experiencing this <u>symptom</u>. The <u>pain</u> in the neck is widespread in people with cervical spinal stenosis. This pain occurs when the spinal canal begins shrinking. The development of bone spurs in elderly individuals with osteoarthritis is a major cause of cervical

Don't Fall!
I'm Falling but, I'm getting up!

stenosis. These spurs compress the nerves, resulting in pain or aching near the neck, including the upper back and shoulders. The development of spurs does not guarantee that neck pain will develop, however.

4. Bladder and Bowel Changes
Many people with spinal stenosis experience changes in bladder and bowel movements. A form of spinal stenosis, Cauda Equina syndrome, causes individuals to feel an increased or urgent need to void the bladder or bowels. The condition can also make it difficult to control the muscles responsible for these actions. People with Cauda Equina syndrome also develop lower   back pain that radiates down the leg and may feel numbness around the anus.
5. Leaning Forward
Those with spinal stenosis report that leaning forward is a means of pain relief. This relief occurs because a forward bend removes the pressure that causes pain. However, this alleviation is temporary; once the person takes a different posture or position, the pain gradually returns. The recurring desire to lean forward to

Don't Fall!
I'm Falling but, I'm getting up!

ease lower <u>back pain</u> can be a sign that a serious issue is at play.

6. Waves of Pain
The type of pain spinal stenosis causes varies from person to person. Many report pains that comes in intense and temporary waves that typically last a few hours, though some flare-ups can last for days. A physician may recommend applying a cold pack to the affected area and restricting movement as much as possible when a person with spinal stenosis is experiencing this symptom.

Don't Fall!
I'm Falling but, I'm getting up!

7. Arthritis
Many people with spinal stenosis have <u>arthritis</u>.
Both osteoarthritis and <u>rheumatoid</u> arthritis can affect the spine, and cause <u>pain</u> and inflammation on that can interfere with movement. Though people with arthritis are prone to developing spinal stenosis, early detection can prevent or minimize this eventual decline. People who experience long-lasting stiffness or pain in the joints should see a doctor.

8.Changes in Posture
Posture is a vital element of a healthy spine. In the case of people with spinal stenosis, a shift in posture is a recurring <u>symptom</u>. As the condition progresses, many people require crutches and braces to walk. Bone spurs that impact the nerves in the spinal cord cause this sign. Posture issues can also lead to <u>sleep</u> quality as people are forced to lie in awkward positions to alleviate <u>pain</u>.

Don't Fall!
I'm Falling but, I'm getting up!

9. Difficulty Standing Up
Because spinal stenosis causes the nerves in the spinal cord to be compressed, many people find it difficult to keep the back straight, which can make it difficult to move from a seated to standing position, and to stand for prolonged periods. Stiffening and tightening of the muscles around the spinal cord also affect an individual's ability to sit and stand straight, and often cause <u>pain</u>.

10. Pain in the Buttocks
Shooting pain in the buttocks and down the leg is one of the signs of lumbar stenosis and is usually due to compression of the nerves that control the lower part of the body as they exit the spinal canal.

Don't Fall!
I'm Falling but, I'm getting up!

Pain in the buttocks that does not go away may also be indicative of other <u>diseases</u> and should, therefore, be examined and diagnosed by a doctor.
Spinal Stenosis.
<u>https://facty.com/conditions/spinal-stenosis/10-symptoms-of-spinal-stenosis/10/</u>
<u>Spinal Stenosis</u>
By Mika, Faculty Staff   Updated: Jun 04, 2019

Don't Fall!
I'm Falling but, I'm getting up!

Chapter 1 Did you know.

An Aging Nation: Projected Number of Children and Older Adults
https://www.census.gov/library/vi

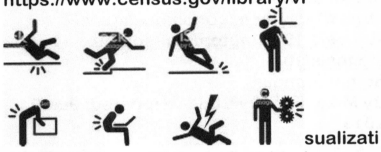

sualizati ons/2018/comm/historic-first.html

Don't Fall!
I'm Falling but, I'm getting up!

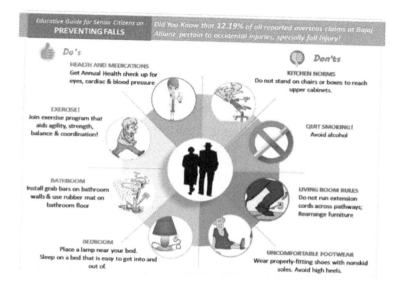

Don't Fall!
I'm Falling but, I'm getting up!

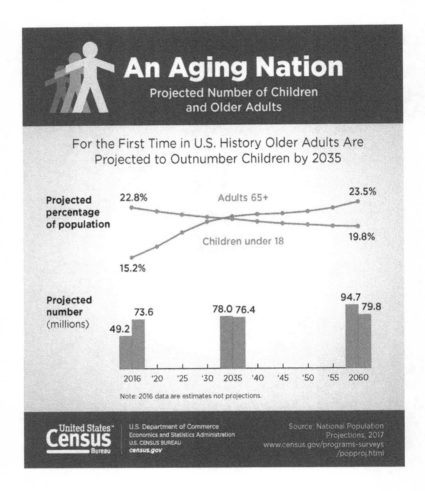

Don't Fall!
I'm Falling but, I'm getting up!

Falls are, unfortunately, a Common Occurrence.
Falls are a serious health issue among seniors. While falls in the general population usually come about due to dangerous work or leisure activities, seniors are at greater risk of falling in their day-to-day activities. Medications, vision impairments, and general weakness can combine with environmental factors to put seniors in danger of seriously injuring themselves in any fall.
11
Every 11 seconds, an older adult is treated in the emergency room for a fall
65
According to the National Council on Aging, one in four Americans over the age of 65 falls each year.
In 2014, older Americans experienced 29 million falls, resulting in
7 million injuries.
19
Every 19 minutes, an older adult die from a fall https://www.aging.com/falls-fact-sheet/

Don't Fall!
I'm Falling but, I'm getting up!

"Awareness of Falls is our best defense
Fall Safety Education
Prevention of Falls

Don't Fall!
I'm Falling but, I'm getting up!

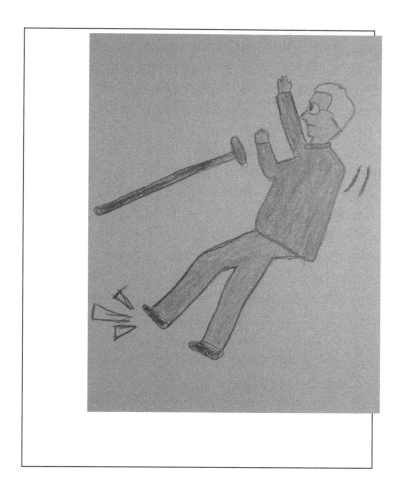

When looking to identify and address fall hazards in any working environment, it is important to understand the different

Don't Fall!
I'm Falling but, I'm getting up!

types of falls that a worker may face while performing their daily tasks.

Falls can be categorized into three types: falls on a single level, falls to a lower level, and swing falls. In this week's post we'll examine these three types of falls and how understanding your workplace fall hazards can help you select the proper fall protection system.

Falls on a Single Level

Falls that occur while a worker remains on a single working level are classified as "slips and falls" or sometimes "slips and trips." Trips result from footways that are uneven, have curved surfaces, or are encroached by fixtures or equipment. Slips can also be a result of the materials coating the footway, for example ice or grease. Worn footwear, or <u>footwear</u> tread that is not matched to the footway can also result in a slip.

In some work environments the fall protection solution for slips and falls may be a simple safety management control, such as maintaining clear footways or specifying footwear tread. But in applications where safety management controls are not enough, fall hazards can be addressed using passive fall protection

Don't Fall!
I'm Falling but, I'm getting up!

systems such as a handrails, catwalks, or enclosed ladders.

Falls to a Lower Level

Most workplace fatalities and serious fall-related injuries result from falls from an elevated level to a lower level. Examples of falls to a lower level include workers falling from mezzanines or from the top of vehicles. Occupational Safety and Health Administration (OSHA) regulations require employers to provide fall protection for workers in any General Industry setting where a worker may fall 4 feet or more to a lower level.

OSHA also requires that active fall protection systems stop a fall to zero acceleration within a distance of 3.5 feet (see OSHA 1915.159). An active fall protection system, such as a full-body harness secured to an overhead anchorage point by means of a self-retracting lanyard (SRL), is likely the best choice for areas where workers risk significant injury or death due to falls from a height.

Swing Falls

Swing falls can also be categorized as a

Don't Fall!
I'm Falling but, I'm getting up!

fall to a lower level, but these types of falls are unique. Swing falls occur when a worker falls from an elevated platform while attached to a fall arrest system and the location of a system's attachment point is not directly over the worker's head. Because the attachment point is not directly overhead, the lanyard the worker is using creates an angle.
During a free fall, this angle of the lanyard causes the worker to swing back towards the attachment point. This may not be a problem if they are falling into open space, but workers are almost always working on top of an object and contact with the object during the swing is inevitable.

Swing falls are commonly encountered in industrial settings such as aircraft manufacturing or maintenance. They can result in fatality, serious injury, or significant damage to equipment.

Swing falls can be prevented by ensuring that workers always tie off to an attachment point and that the attachment point always remains overhead.

Don't Fall!
I'm Falling but, I'm getting up!

Identifying the fall risks in a work environment is essential in choosing the most appropriate fall protection system. Once identified, managers and employers can design and <u>purchase</u> a system tailored to the specific needs of their facility.
<u>https://www.rigidlifelines.com/blog/entry/three-types-of-workplace-falls#</u>

Don't Fall!
I'm Falling but, I'm getting up!

Chapter 3 Facts on Falls.

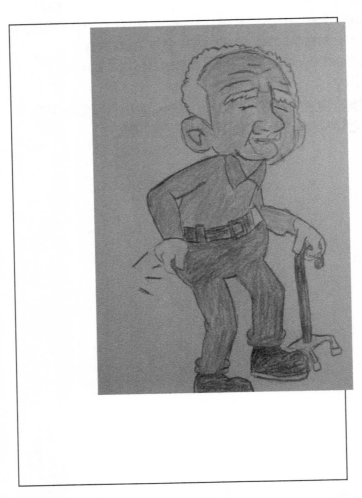

The Most Important Stats & Facts About Falls in the Elderly

Don't Fall!
I'm Falling but, I'm getting up!

Falls among the elderly have seen a 31% spike according to a decade-long study.
In 2014 alone, falls accounted for 7 million injuries in 29 million seniors in the US.
Elderly individuals 65 years and older suffer the most deaths from falls.
One senior fall fatality occurs every 19 minutes.
In both the US and the UK, falls are the most reported incidents in hospitals.
Every 11 seconds, there's an elderly person receiving emergency care for a fall.
Around the globe, 37.3 million fall incidents result in serious injuries yearly.
Over 95% of accidents in seniors cause debilitating hip fractures.
A traumatic brain injury occurs in 79% of elderly fall cases.
When it comes to inpatient falls, hospitals are viewed as 100% legally accountable.

Don't Fall!
I'm Falling but, I'm getting up!

What Causes Falls?

1. Several falls statistics reveal that bad weather, glare from bright lights, clutter, or even recently rearranged furniture can contribute to a higher fall risk. (Aging.com)
Storms (or just plain, old rainy weather) and failing to keep up with household maintenance may cause leaks, making it more likely to slip inside the home. Unorganized spaces, areas cluttered by obstacles like storage boxes and out-of-place cords, and furnishings placed where people walk all represent some danger. Relatives and senior caretakers should keep an eye out for these kinds of safety hazards. The Canadian Centre for Occupational Health and Safety (CCOHS) found that 67% of falls aren't ones that happen from a height, but rather are same-level ones where individuals slipped or tripped.

Don't Fall!
I'm Falling but, I'm getting up!

2. In the case of elderly falls,
the facts show that as people age, they're
more susceptible to sustaining broken
bones after a fall.
(National Institutes of Health)
This is a grave problem. According to the
National Institutes of Health, broken
bones are linked to osteoporosis. And
according to the Mayo Clinic,
osteoporosis is a disease that impedes
bone tissue regeneration. As a result, the
bones become weak and brittle—when
viewed under a microscope, these bones
appear more porous, with bigger "holes"
than normal (the name literally means
"porous bone").

The condition can get so severe that a
violent cough alone may result in a bone
fracture. Symptoms include height loss, a
slouching posture due to the spine
curving, and back pain. Oftentimes, many
people aren't aware that they
have osteoporosis in the first place, which
is in part why the disease is so dangerous,
especially in older persons.

Don't Fall!
I'm Falling but, I'm getting up!

3. Stats on older adults and falls mention that ill-fitting clothing and shoes, or impractical footwear, also contribute to a higher likelihood of falling.
(Aging.com)

Seems like an obscure thought that shouldn't need any further explanation, but the Illinois Podiatric Medical Association (IPMA) cites that 75% of people in the US will experience foot problems at least once in their lifetime.

Just think about it for a moment. How many hours a day do we spend on our feet, <u>mobile</u> or standing stationary? The IPMA answers this question creatively with an interesting fact: Did you know that a 70-year-old will have walked so much in their lifetime that the distance they cover would be the equivalent of a stroll around the world?

Not just one trip, but four times around the globe, apparently. It's important to keep these falls in the elderly statistics in mind when purchasing our clothing and footwear.

Don't Fall!
I'm Falling but, I'm getting up!

4. Ear disorders affect balance and are among the additional conditions that can increase one's chances of taking a fall. (Aging.com)
The ears play a crucial part in the way the body balances itself. The movement of fluid in the ears' semicircular canals work together with sail-like structures called the cupulae to send head movement signals to the brain. This is why ear infections and stuffiness from colds tend to make people dizzy and unstable on their feet.

Additionally, there's an actual condition relating to imbalance that occurs in 35% of Americans 40 years of age and older. The condition, called inner ear balance disorder, is described as "a vestibular dysfunction of the inner ear" by WebMD.

The 2009 article reports that individuals who displayed symptoms of the disorder were more likely to experience a fall of some kind. Statistics of falls in the elderly reveal this to be eight times more likely, in fact. What's worse, it seems that the disorder typically presents itself in older age groups. With a host of ear-

Don't Fall!
I'm Falling but, I'm getting up!

related issues potentially causing balance problems, it's critical that elderly individuals undergo checkups on a regular basis.

5. Medical conditions such as Parkinson's <u>disease</u> and kidney problems may increase the risk of falls.
(Wisconsin State Journal)

The European Parkinson's Disease Association (EPDA) goes over several reasons why falls are associated with the disease. Firstly, though, they clarify that not all individuals with Parkinson's are automatically susceptible to fall incidents.

However, the disease affects the nervous system and movement, which is why these statistics about falls in the elderly indicate that it brings a greater risk.

Oftentimes, it begins with tremors or stiffness. Changes to an individual's posture, weakening muscles, low blood pressure, <u>eye problems</u>, instability, and a freezing gait are all symptoms. These symptoms occur because dopamine

Don't Fall!
I'm Falling but, I'm getting up!

levels dwindle and tend to become worse as time passes, and they render falls more likely.
6. Medications such as sedatives and antidepressants also contribute to an increased fall risk in older individuals. (Aging.com)

One reason for this is because medications tend to have stronger effects among the elderly than in younger individuals. Drugs that slow the heart rate or lower <u>blood pressure</u> are also one of the many culprits that may lead to hypotension or syncope, and eventually a fall.

Analysis of elderly falls statistics and medications have revealed that discontinuing cardiovascular medications reduces the chances of a tumble by half. The CDC warns that even seemingly harmless over-the-counter medicines can increase the risk of falls.

7. According to the Agency for Healthcare Research and Quality, analgesics, opiates, antipsychotics, and

Don't Fall!
I'm Falling but, I'm getting up!

anticonvulsants are all medicines that cause a high fall risk.
(Geriatrics Medicine)
Psychotropics such as antidepressants can result in low sodium levels and, in turn, gait and attention issues that can induce falls. Anti-anxiety medications, on the other hand, may produce the same side effects as above, but they can also cause psychomotor dysfunctions, drug dependence, and even delirium.

8. Hearing loss has also been linked to a higher risk of falls in older people, as the statistics compiled in a 2015 review show.

(Healthy Hearing)
We've discussed how the ears play a key part in transmitting signals to the brain to maintain positioning and balance. As it turns out, it isn't just ear infections that impede the ear's ability to play this role. A study from the Johns Hopkins School of Medicine found that even with mild hearing loss, elderly participants had three times the risk of experiencing a fall. And to make matters worse, the risk

Don't Fall!
I'm Falling but, I'm getting up!

increases by 140% with every 10 decibels of hearing range shrinkage.
Fortunately, the study also made a significant discovery: hearing aids counter the negative effects that hearing loss has on balance. This has led researchers to conclude that auditory cues play a significant part in spatial awareness, similar to how the eyes affect balance when lights in a room are suddenly turned off.

9. Statistics on falls in the elderly indicate a positive correlation between fat in the midsection and an increased fall risk. (Harvard Health)
The study, published in the American Journal of Preventive Medicine, included fall histories spanning two years from seniors 65 years old and over. Data was gathered from a sample of about 3,400 elderly individuals. It found that those with central obesity were 37% more likely to experience a fall than those who had low to no visceral fat. Scientists reason that a higher center of gravity for obese individuals is probably a major factor to instability. (The lower the center of gravity, the more stable something is.)

Don't Fall!
I'm Falling but, I'm getting up!

Informative Facts and Statistics on Elderly Falls

10. The one-year mortality rate in seniors over 60 is as high as 58% following injuries related to trips, slips, and falls, statistics in the elderly show.
(MKInjury)
As you read through the previous section and learned about the causes of falls in the elderly, you may have noticed something critical: many of the causes are easily associated with aging.

From hearing loss to sensitivity to medication, the human body undergoes changes that wind up making seniors the most at-risk demographic for falls and related injuries. Even a perfectly healthy senior without pre-existing conditions has a higher risk of falling than an individual from a younger age group simply because of how age affects the body.

11. As for falls and their treatment in hospitals, statistics reveal that there's an elderly person receiving treatment for a fall every 11 seconds in the emergency room.

Don't Fall!
I'm Falling but, I'm getting up!

(Aging.com)
The range of injuries from falls can be something as harmless as a minor cut or bruise to a severe disability, and sometimes death. The level of physical damage from a fall depends on the energy the body absorbs on impact. Whether or not an individual sustains an injury depends on several factors: how they land, how strong their bones are, how their tissues absorb the energy of the impact, and how well their neuromuscular reflexes react to lessen the impact.

12. Patient falls in hospitals, according to statistics, occur in 700,000 to 1 million patients yearly.
(Patient Safety Network)
Studies have gone on to reveal that for every 1,000 days spent in the hospital, fall events occur at a rate of 3–5 times. The prevalence is higher among elderly patients, and of the injuries that take place from these fall incidents, one-third are serious. Because patient safety is considered basic protection and falls are regarded as easily preventable, patient falls are considered "never events" and therefore aren't covered by Medicare and

Don't Fall!
I'm Falling but, I'm getting up!

Medicaid. https://medalerthelp.org/falls-in-the-elderly-statistics/

Although people of all ages experience falls, seniors are at particular risk of falls, including falls that result in potentially serious, even life-altering injuries. The Centers for Disease Control and Prevention (CDC) reports that one in four seniors' experiences at least one fall every year.

One in five falls among seniors result in serious injuries, such as broken bones or head injuries. Other statistics related to falls among seniors show that more than three million seniors receive treatment at emergency departments every year due to a fall and that 800,000 individuals are admitted to the hospital after experiencing a fall.

Advancing age plays a significant role in falls among seniors. Seniors that are 75 years of age and older that fall are five times more likely to be admitted to a long-term care facility for at least a year, compared to younger seniors, aged 65 through 74 years of age.

Don't Fall!
I'm Falling but, I'm getting up!

13. Additional falls in the hospital statistics demonstrate that most tumbles occur in the bathroom or by the patient's bed.
(U.S. National Library of Medicine)
These types of falls tend to happen among patients experiencing a state of confusion or physical instability. The prevalence of these reported falls seems to be increasing. This is likely due to a variety of reasons, such as better reporting systems, nurses having less time to spend with each patient, and a rising number of older patients receiving care—not to mention the increased number of patients who are seriously ill or under heavy sedation.

14. In the case of patient falls, statistics show that they're preventable, meaning the fault is considered to lie solely with the hospital.
(Van Wey, Presby, & Williams Law)
Fall prevention in hospitals is considered a basic responsibility and part of the hospital's duty in providing care. Updated standards in patient care require that hospitals assess patients in their care for fall risk. They're also held responsible for

Don't Fall!
I'm Falling but, I'm getting up!

managing risk factors like environmental hazards, medical conditions, and certain fall-inducing side effects from medications such as drowsiness and confusion.

15. Patient falls statistics from 2015 through 2016 alone revealed that falls are the most reported incident among both acute and community hospitals in the United Kingdom.
(National Health Service)
For mental health hospitals, falls ranked third on the "most reported incidents" list. Analyzing inpatient falls data in England, the report found that overall around 250,000 falls were reported in that particular year alone. It goes on to reveal that community hospitals have the highest falls per 1,000 bed days. Since elderly patients tend to stay at community hospitals for long periods due to a slower recovery, they're at a higher risk for falling, potentially even falling several times.

16. In the United States, accidental falls in older people are shown by statistics to be the most reported incident at hospitals.

Don't Fall!
I'm Falling but, I'm getting up!

(U.S. National Library of Medicine)
Data from the National Database of Nursing Quality Indicators (NDNQI) showed that fall rates vary per nursing unit type. Medical nursing units tended to have the highest fall rates and the highest number of injury-sustaining falls despite having healthier older patients. This is attributed to these elderly individuals being more mobile. This, in turn, puts them in more situations where they might fall.

17. Every year, 37.3 million cases of falls worldwide result in serious injuries that need medical treatment.
(World Health Organization)
These particular instances result in over 17 million disability-adjusted life years (DALYs) lost, as reflected in many falls in the elderly statistics. For clarification, a single DALY is defined by the WHO as "one lost year of healthy life." High morbidity from falls mostly occurs in people 65 years old and above and in children at the age of 15 or younger. Recent data suggests that 40% of lost DALYs are from falls in children. There is suspicion, however, that DALYs in older

Don't Fall!
I'm Falling but, I'm getting up!

age groups are inaccurate since, for starters, they have fewer life years to account for.

18. Additional statistics for falls in the elderly from the WHO reveal that seniors above 65 suffer the most fatalities.
(World Health Organization)
In their 2018 fact sheet, the World Health Organization (WHO) explained that groups with the highest risk for falls are elderly individuals and children. They also disclosed that fatality rates in seniors increase with age. In the US, up to 30% of falls incur injuries, from bruising to head trauma and hip fractures. In children, falls happen mostly because kids, as they grow and develop, tend to test their independence, become more curious, and wind up taking more risks.

19. The elderly fall stats show that from 2007 to 2016 the incidence rate of falls has been a rising trend, with a 31% increase overall.
(American Physical Therapy Association)
This 10-year study conducted by the CDC reveals that fatal falls have risen from 18,334 to 29,668 among Americans 65

Don't Fall!
I'm Falling but, I'm getting up!

years old and above, with a climb rate of approximately 3% per year. There's also a variance between states. For example, the gap between Wisconsin and Alabama is especially huge, the death rates being 142.7 per 100,000 and 24.4 per 100,000 persons, respectively.

These statistics on elderly falls in the US may vary due to the inconsistent distribution of certain age-based demographics. The numbers may also be skewed by medical reports, since for some reason coroners tend to designate falls as the cause of death 14% less often than medical examiners.

Don't Fall!
I'm Falling but, I'm getting up!

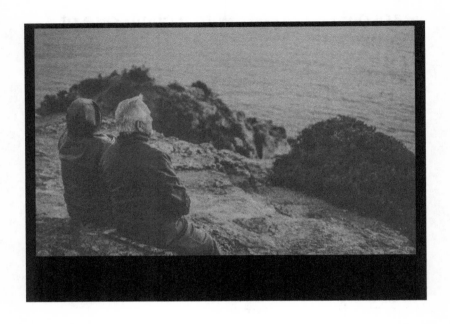

20. There were 7 million injuries from falls among 29 million elderly Americans in 2014.
(Aging.com)
The following year didn't just see an increase in falls among older age groups in the United States. There was also $50 billion in costs as part of
the consequences of falls in the elderly. 75% was shouldered by Medicare and Medicaid.

Don't Fall!
I'm Falling but, I'm getting up!

According to the CDC, 20% of falls result in a serious injury, which is a direct contributor to these costs, sometimes leading to medical bankruptcy. It isn't the falls themselves that pose long-term risks and costs, but the related injuries that occur. In elderly people taking medications like blood thinners, for example, the seriousness of injuries and complications are even more dire. Blood thinners can be lifesaving, but for those who experience a fall, they can worsen those injuries by causing excessive bleeding and bone fractures.

21. According to the slips, trips, and falls statistics from 2019, over 95% of these accidents in the elderly result in hip fractures.
(MKInjury)
Hip fractures can occur in the elderly who suffer from osteoarthritis, and the often involve surgery or hip replacement. Along with that comes a long recovery period with physical therapy. It can take anywhere from six months to an entire year for recovery, and during this extended period, physicians recommend

Don't Fall!
I'm Falling but, I'm getting up!

minimizing pivoting or twisting movements along the leg and hip. Naturally, this dominoes into other issues: loss of independence and insecurity moving around. Plus, the physical inactivity may result in even more complications such as bed sores, a urinary tract infection, muscle atrophy, blood clots, and depression.

22. In 2013, falls accounted for nearly 50% of traumatic brain injury (TBI) cases in hospitals.
(PennyGeeks)
Within the elderly population, these senior fall facts revealed a whopping 79% TBI incidence rate. This type of injury is especially dangerous since at first, patients may seem completely fine. On impact, the nerve fibers may tear, in addition to bruising in the brain. Trauma is often delayed, but eventually, swelling can push the brain against the skull, significantly decreasing blood flow.
Fluid buildup causes intracranial pressure as the brain tries to repair itself, which can cause further damage to other parts of the brain. Depending on the injury's severity, a blood vessel may rupture and

Don't Fall!
I'm Falling but, I'm getting up!

result in a blood clot that produces added pressure yet again. Unfortunately, seniors 75 years of age and older are the most vulnerable to traumatic brain injuries and, ultimately, to the resulting TBI fatalities.

23. CDC fall statistics also reveal that falls account for 95% of hip fractures in the 300,000 elderly people who end up being hospitalized for it per year.
(The Journal)
The American Family Physician asserts that 25% of seniors who wind up falling and fracturing their hip die within six months of sustaining the injury. More than 50% of seniors who recover from hip fractures end up in nursing homes. And of these, another half remain in nursing homes for another year. This is in large part because the road to recovery from this type of injury is often littered with complications, including catheter-associated urinary tract infections or pressure ulcers from being immobile for longer periods of time.

24. In the aging population, a major cause of death is senior falls, with one death by fall occurring every 19 minutes.

Don't Fall!
I'm Falling but, I'm getting up!

(Aging.com)
In fact, falls are the primary cause of both non-fatal and fatal trauma in seniors. The National Council on Aging purports that 25% of Americans above 65 years of age experience falls yearly. Emergency facilities also treat more than 2.8 million cases a year due to falls. Of these cases, more than 800,000 result in hospital confinement and over 27,000 in death.

25. In the UK, falls in older people were shown in statistics to account for 77% of the total falls reported by hospitals. (National Health Service)
These falls, however, accounted for a whopping 87% share of the actual associated costs. Of the £2.3 billion nationwide total that accounted for costs from falls both inside and outside of hospitals, elderly falls made up 25%. Experts at the NHS extrapolated that a facility with beds for 800 patients will have about 1,500 falls, meaning £1.9 million. This doesn't even account for every expenditure. The estimate doesn't include external costs like the price of rehabilitation services outside of hospitals

Don't Fall!
I'm Falling but, I'm getting up!

and the need for assisted care facility stays, for example.

26. The National Council on Aging forecasts that hip fractures due to falls will rise by 12% by 2030.
(The Journal)
This increase and the overall rising trend in elderly falls statistics likely correlates with an increased aging population worldwide. Due to the decline in fertility and increased longevity because of better living standards, the share of the elderly among the global population is increasing. According to the United Nations, developing regions will house 79% of the world's population of seniors 60 years of age and older by 2050. More importantly, the study, spanning 143 countries, also found that in countries like the Netherlands, the prevalence of seniors 60 and over who live independently was as high as 93.4%.

27. Annually, around 9,500 senior fatalities are attributed to falls.
(The Journal)
There's a direct correlation between falls in the elderly and mortality. Among older

Don't Fall!
I'm Falling but, I'm getting up!

age groups, falls are the primary cause of fatal and non-fatal trauma. And it isn't just the fall and resulting injuries that are a cause of concern. Trips to the ER typically mean a long period of recovery and vulnerability afterward. It's during these periods that sharp declines in health occur because usually elderly individuals will still attempt to do things themselves even though they're not fully recovered.

28. For seniors, fall statistics from 2019 reveal Wisconsin as the state with the highest rate of deadly falls in the United States.
(Wisconsin State Journal)
In Wisconsin, 27% of deadly falls in seniors happened at a care facility of some kind, based on 2015–2017 data. In 2017, 2,664 falls were reported by assisted living facilities—even higher than 2016's 2,371 reported falls. According to the Centers for Medicare and Medicaid, Wisconsin's fall rate among the elderly in nursing homes is 19.6%—higher than the national average, which is 17%. Wisconsin's number of citations per nursing home facility is also higher than the national average, at 130 citations in

Don't Fall!
I'm Falling but, I'm getting up!

2018. This information is based on data studied by Jim Robinson, a senior scientist at the University of Wisconsin's Center for Health Systems and Research Analysis.
Elderly Fall Prevention

29. Keeping hospital pathways clear of obstructions such as medical equipment helps reduce patient falls.
(Medline Plus)
Patients in recovery tend to get easily disoriented due to weakness and instability. If a fall occurs, it's important that hospital staff report the incident, evaluate the patient for injuries, check for alertness, and keep a close eye on them. If the patient can be safely moved, a healthcare professional should assist them back to bed or into a wheelchair with the help of another staff member. Nevertheless, prevention is the best way to protect patients. Statistics of falls in the elderly show that keeping floors from being slippery and using good lighting are simple but effective measures in fall prevention.

Don't Fall!
I'm Falling but, I'm getting up!

30. Hospital patient falls statistics show that recent projects in fall prevention have actually been effective, resulting in a 35% reduction of hospital fall rates.
(The Joint Commission Center for Transforming Healthcare)
These projects also reduced the rate of falls that led to an injury by an impressive 63%. The Preventing Falls Targeting Solutions Tool, a "fact-based, systematic and data-driven problem-solving approach," brought this about. Using a Six Sigma Lean approach, the Joint Commission developed the process to help facilities reduce falls. This approach—formed after thoughtful research into the pertinent elderly falls facts and data—is designed to achieve a "zero harm" or "no falls" status.

31. For elderly people coping with Parkinson's disease, the EPDA names attentional strategies and visual and rhythmical cues as tools that help reduce the likelihood of falls.
(The European Parkinson's Disease Association)
The European Parkinson's Disease Association (EPDA) explains that these

cues are helpful because they use the part of the brain that's unaffected by the disease. With visual cues, for example, an individual can use lines on the ground or patterns on the floor to help stabilize movement and keep their steps uniform while walking. Steady rhythms from music or a metronome also help achieve a similar effect.

32. Among other measures, the WHO recommends consulting with healthcare professionals to assess risk factors for falls.
(World Health Organization)
An earlier section discussed falls in the elderly statistics and the factors that contribute to increased chances of falls. A considerable number of them were medical conditions like low blood pressure, low blood sodium, ear infections, and any others that can cause dizziness or syncope. A doctor will be able to screen for these as well as evaluate any medications that make a fall more likely.

33. The WHO also suggests that at-risk elderly individuals participate in Tai-Chi

Don't Fall!
I'm Falling but, I'm getting up!

and similar exercises for strength training and balance development to fight off falls. (World Health Organization)

Harvard Health offers new senior fall facts asserting that Tai Chi has many health benefits for the elderly when it comes to fall prevention. As a slow and deliberate form of exercise, it promotes confidence in physical movement. Due to this approach, it can help overcome the fear of falling down again, which is crucial. For many seniors, this fear actually increases the likelihood of future falls.

It also hones proprioception—the sense of positional bodily awareness—a key element in promoting balance.

Additionally, without pain or overexertion, practitioners can build muscular strength and flexibility. Dr. Gloria Yeh, an assistant professor at Harvard Medical School, explains that the controlled, unsupported movements in Tai Chi work the body's core muscles, as well as the lower and upper extremities.

34. Devices with fall detection technology are now on the market to help seniors should they suffer a fall.

Don't Fall!
I'm Falling but, I'm getting up!

(Apple Insider)
The falls in elderly statistics didn't fall on deaf ears—there are many medical alert systems and other devices that offer fall detection out there. Even tech giants like Apple are taking an interest. Here's how the feature works: using built-in sensors, the Apple Watch Series 4 detects swift movements that indicate the wearer may have had a fall. It issues alerts, then if the wearer remains immobile for a long period of time and doesn't respond to the message alerts, it contacts emergency services.

According to Apple Insider, in the case of 67-year-old Toralv Ostvang, his Series 4 contacting Emergency Services undoubtedly saved his life. He was discovered unconscious in his home in Norway when the response team arrived. Later tests revealed he suffered multiple skull fractures that would have probably resulted in death if emergency care hadn't been administered.

35. The CDC, to combat falls in hospitals, created the STEADI program,

Don't Fall!
I'm Falling but, I'm getting up!

which provides a better quality of life and shortens hospital stays.
(Centers for Disease Control and Prevention)

The program promotes the screening of older individuals for fall risk factors. It then identifies and works on reducing the ones that can be mitigated. After a two-year study of the program, researchers found that its implementation reduced the average length of hospital stays from 7.9 to 6.5 days. Of the discharged patients, nearly 10% more were discharged home. Before STEADI, 1.5% of patients who suffered a fall returned for treatment for another fall. This number was reduced to 0.6%.

FAQ

High Risk of falling?
When you see patients 65 and older, make these three questions a routine part of your exam:
Have you fallen in the past year?
Do you feel unsteady when standing or walking?

Don't Fall!
I'm Falling but, I'm getting up!

Do you worry about falling?
If your patient answers "yes" to any of these key screening questions, they are considered at increased risk of falling. Further assessment is recommended. Seniors are at high risk for serious falls As we age, our <u>bodies change</u>. These gradual changes add up to increased fall risk for older adults.

With age may come wisdom and, all too frequently, a fall. Falls are common causes of serious injuries. One out of every three people over 65 falls every year in the U.S. And that fall may be the last. In 1995, a fall was fatal to nearly 8,000 Americans over 65.
What Conditions Make You More Likely to Fall?

Research has identified many conditions that contribute to falling. These are called risk factors. Many risk factors can be changed or modified to help prevent falls. They include:
Lower body weakness
Vitamin D deficiency (that is, not enough vitamin D in your system)
Difficulties with walking and balance

Don't Fall!
I'm Falling but, I'm getting up!

Use of medicines, such as tranquilizers, sedatives, or antidepressants. Even some over-the-counter medicines can affect balance and how steady you are on your feet.

Vision problems
Foot pain or poor footwear
Home hazards or dangers such as broken or uneven steps, and
throw rugs or clutter that can be tripped over.

Most falls are caused by a combination of risk factors. The more risk factors a person has, the greater their chances of falling.
Healthcare providers can help cut down a person's risk by reducing the fall risk factors listed above.
What medical factors increase the chance of a fall?

Medical factors that contribute to falls among seniors include:
Visual impairment, such as
from myopia or cataracts;
Disorders of the nervous system, such as sciatica;

74

Don't Fall!
I'm Falling but, I'm getting up!

Joint and muscle problems, such as occur with <u>arthritis</u>;
Difficulties in gait and balance, such as in <u>Parkinson'</u> <u>disease</u>; a dedications which induce sleepiness.

Don't Fall!
I'm Falling but, I'm getting up!

Chapter 4 Myths.

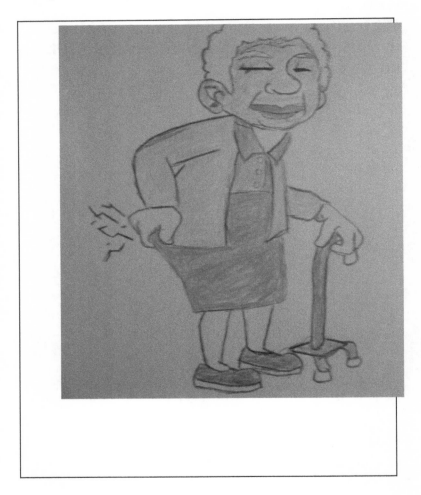

Don't Fall!
I'm Falling but, I'm getting up!

Older Adults (debunking the Myths Older Adults Falls) National Council on Aging

Myth 1: Falling happens to other people, not to me.
Reality: Many people think, "It won't happen to me." But the truth is that 1 in 4 older adults <u>fall every year</u> in the U.S.

Myth 2: Falling is something normal that happens as you get older.
Reality: Falling is not a normal part of aging. Strength and balance exercises, managing your medications, having your vision checked and making your living environment safer are all steps you can take to prevent a fall.

Myth 3: If I limit my activity, I won't fall.
Reality: Some people believe that the best way to prevent falls is to stay at home and limit activity. Not true. Performing physical activities will actually help you stay independent, as your strength and range of motion benefit from remaining active. Social activities are also good for your overall health.

Don't Fall!
I'm Falling but, I'm getting up!

Myth 4: As long as I stay at home, I can avoid falling.
Reality: Over half of all falls take place at home. Inspect your home for fall risks. Fix simple but serious hazards such as clutter, throw rugs, and poor lighting. Make simple home modifications, such as adding grab bars in the bathroom, a second handrail on stairs, and non-slip paint on outdoor steps.

Myth 5: Muscle strength and flexibility can't be regained.
Reality: While we do lose muscle as we age, exercise can partially restore strength and flexibility. It's never too late to start an exercise program. Even if you've been a "couch potato" your whole life, becoming active now will benefit you in many ways—including protection from falls.

Myth 6: Taking medication doesn't increase my risk of falling.
Reality: Taking any medication may increase your risk of falling. Medications affect people in many different ways and can sometimes make you dizzy or sleepy. Be careful when starting a new

Don't Fall!
I'm Falling but, I'm getting up!

medication. Talk to your <u>health care</u> <u>provider</u> about potential side effects or interactions of your medications.

Myth 7: I don't need to get my vision checked every year.
Reality: Vision is another key risk factor for falls. Aging is associated with some forms of vision loss that increase risk of falling and injury. People with vision problems are more than twice as likely to fall as those without visual impairment. Have your eyes checked at least once a year and update your eyeglasses. For those with low vision there are programs and assistive devices that can help. Ask your optometrist for a referral.

Myth 8: Using a walker or cane will make me more dependent.
Reality: Walking aids are very important in helping many older adults maintain or improve their mobility. However, make sure you use these devices safely. Have a physical therapist fit the walker or cane to you and instruct you in its safe use.

Myth 9: I don't need to talk to family <u>members</u> or my health care

Don't Fall!
I'm Falling but, I'm getting up!

provider if I'm concerned about my risk of falling. I don't want to alarm them, and I want to keep my independence.
Reality: Fall prevention is a team effort. Bring it up with your doctor, family, and anyone else who is in a position to help. They want to help you maintain your mobility and reduce your risk of falling.

Myth 10: I don't need to talk to my parent, spouse, or other older adult if I'm concerned about their risk of falling. It will hurt their feelings, and it's none of my business.

Reality: Let them know about your concerns and offer support to help them maintain the highest degree of independence possible. There are many things you can do, including removing hazards in the home, finding a fall prevention program in the community, or setting up a vision exam.
https://www.ncoa.org/healthy-aging/falls-prevention/preventing-falls-tips-for-older-adults-and-caregivers/debunking-the-myths-of-older-adult-falls/

Don't Fall!
I'm Falling but, I'm getting up!

Chapter 5 What you need to know (to do) after a Fall.

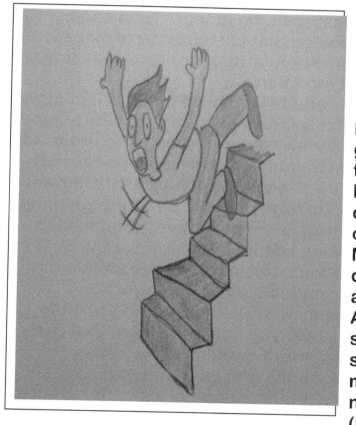

Right kind of Medical Assessment (Be Proactive)

Don't Fall!
I'm Falling but, I'm getting up!

Be proactive about getting the right kind
of medical assessment after a fall. Why?
There are three major reasons for this:
A fall can be a sign of a new and serious
medical problem that needs treatment.
For instance, an older person can be
weakened and fall because of illnesses
such as dehydration, or a serious urinary
tract infection.
Older adults who have fallen are at higher
risk for a future fall. Although it's a good
idea for any older person to be proactive
about identifying and reducing fall risk
factors, it's vital to do this well after a fall.
Busy doctors may not be thorough unless
caregivers are proactive about asking
questions. Most doctors have the best
intentions, but studies have shown that
older patients often don't get
recommended care. By being politely
proactive, you can make sure that certain
things aren't overlooked (such as
medications that worsen balance).
All too often, a medical visit after a fall is
mainly about addressing any injuries that
the older person may have suffered.
Obviously, this is very important!
However, if you want to help prevent
future falls, it's also important to make

Don't Fall!
I'm Falling but, I'm getting up!

sure the doctors have checked on all the things that could have contributed to the fall.

Always assess injuries before moving! If you find that your older adult has been injured in a fall, don't move them – that could make their injuries worse. Instead, call 911, keep them as warm and comfortable as possible, and wait for emergency responders to arrive.

Essential tips After a Fall
Stay calm and don't move for a few minutes. Moving too quickly can cause more harm.

Figure out if anything was injured. Slowly move hands and feet, arms and legs.

Assuming there are no injuries, slowly roll onto your side. Rest a little.

Slowly push up into a crawling position and crawl slowly toward a sturdy chair or furniture item. Don't rush. Rest as needed. Put one hand at a time on the seat of the chair.

Supporting yourself with the chair, bring your strongest leg up to a 90-degree angle by putting that foot flat on the ground. The other leg stays in kneeling position.

Don't Fall!
I'm Falling but, I'm getting up!

Slowly push up to standing using both arms and legs.
Slowly turn around and lower yourself onto the chair.
Sit and catch your breath for a few minutes before doing anything else.

A True Story:
Re: https://www.webmd.com/healthy-aging/features/falling-injuries-preventable#1
Eleanor Kusel never gave much consideration to the bumps in the sidewalks or the rugs lying on the floor of her apartment. But after the 75-year-old San Franciscan fell and fractured her pelvis while getting out of a car, she began to notice the many hazards that could cause her to fall again.
"I never thought about it until this happened," Kusel said of her recent accident.
Kusel is not alone. One out of every three Americans 65 years and older falls at least once a year, with 10 percent fracturing a bone, dislocating Mary Tinetti, Chief of Geriatrics at the Yale University School of Medicine.

Don't Fall!
I'm Falling but, I'm getting up!

After three months of bed rest and therapy, Kusel is gradually moving back into her daily routine. She's resumed her volunteer work at a local hospital and is once again making her way around town.

While common sense dictates that falling accidents are the result of household hazards such as slippery bathroom floors or poorly lit stairwells, that's not what some researchers have found.

In a recent study, Yale University researchers identified hazards in the homes of 1,100 people who were 72 years or older. After following the study participants for three years, the researchers compared the number of falls with the kinds of household hazards they initially identified. The result: household hazards did not affect the number of falls people had.

https://dailycaring.com/video-how-to-safely-get-up-after-a-fall/
https://www.cdc.gov/steadi/patient.html#
https://www.cdc.gov/homeandrecreationalsafety/falls/index.html

What to Do When a Fall Occurs
Falls of Seniors can be Prevented

Don't Fall!
I'm Falling but, I'm getting up!

Intervention
A multicomponent/multifactorial intervention based on individual risk factors should be implemented to help prevent future falls in community-dwelling older persons. Intervention to prevent falls should be considered in older persons living in long-term care facilities, taking into <u>account</u> their physical ability and health status. There is insufficient evidence to recommend for or against intervention in older persons with cognitive impairment.

Don't Fall!
I'm Falling but, I'm getting up!

MEDICATION MODIFICATION
Medications are often associated with increased risk of falling. The strongest evidence for reducing this risk supports withdrawal of psychotropic medications (e.g., sedative hypnotics, anxiolytics, antidepressants, antipsychotics). Dosage reduction is an <u>option</u> in patients who cannot stop taking a medication because of a medical condition. Minimizing the number of medications, a patient is taking should be considered in older persons at increased risk of falling.

EXERCISE
All patients should be offered an exercise program that includes strength training and balance and gait exercises, such as tai chi and physical therapy. Flexibility and endurance training should also be offered as additional exercises. The program should be tailored to the patient's health and physical ability and reviewed regularly. Individual and group exercise programs are equally effective.

VISION IMPAIRMENT
There is insufficient evidence to recommend vision assessment and

Don't Fall!
I'm Falling but, I'm getting up!

intervention to prevent falls in older persons. However, if a patient reports problem with vision, a formal assessment should be performed and any remediable visual abnormalities treated, particularly cataract. Patients should be advised not to wear multifocal lenses while walking.

MANAGEMENT OF POSTURAL HYPOTENSION

Assessment and treatment of postural hypotension should be a component of fall prevention. The condition, which leads to loss of balance, is usually caused by dehydration, concomitant medication use, or autonomic neuropathy.

CARDIOVASCULAR FACTORS

Common cardiovascular disorders associated with falls include carotid sinus hypersensitivity, vasovagal syndrome, bradyarrhythmia's, and tachyarrhythmias. Dual chamber cardiac pacing may be considered for older persons with cardioinhibitory carotid sinus hypersensitivity who have had unexplained, recurrent falls.

Don't Fall!
I'm Falling but, I'm getting up!

VITAMIN D SUPPLEMENTATION
Vitamin D deficiency is common in older persons and can impair muscle strength and neuromuscular function. Supplementation has been shown to be beneficial in preventing falls in older persons with vitamin D deficiency, and possibly in those with normal vitamin D levels. Therefore, vitamin D supplementation (at least 800 IU per day) should be used to treat deficiency and should be considered for all older persons.

MANAGEMENT OF FOOT AND FOOTWEAR PROBLEMS
Foot problems, such as bunions, toe or nail deformities, and ulcers, should be identified and treated to prevent falls in older persons. Poor or improper footwear can also increase the risk of falls, and older persons should be advised to wear shoes with low heels and high surface contact area.

HOME MODIFICATION
A health care professional should assess the patient's home so that it can be modified to reduce or eliminate hazards.

Don't Fall!
I'm Falling but, I'm getting up!

Common home hazards include inadequate lighting, absence of railings, and clutter. Safe performance of activities of daily living also should be promoted.

EDUCATION

Fall prevention programs should include education about risk factors and strategies to minimize risk. Education may include access to resources (e.g., durable medical equipment, local exercise programs) and opportunities to develop fall prevention skills (e.g., practicing safely getting into the bathtub).

Don't Fall!
I'm Falling but, I'm getting up!

CDC Reports

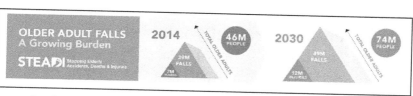

1. An assessment for underlying new illness. Doctors almost always do this if an older person has been having generalized weakness, delirium, or other signs of feeling unwell. Be sure to bring up any symptoms you've noticed, and let the doctor know how quickly the changes came on.

Just about any new health problem that makes an older person weak can bring on a fall. Some common ones include:
Urinary tract infection
Dehydration

Anemia (low red blood cell count), which can be brought on by bleeding in the bowel or by other causes
Pneumonia
Heart problems such as atrial fibrillation

Don't Fall!
I'm Falling but, I'm getting up!

Strokes, including mini strokes that don't cause weakness on one side

2. A blood pressure and pulse reading when sitting, and when standing. This is especially important if you've been worried about falls — or near falls — that are associated with light-headedness, or fainting.

If your older relative takes blood pressure medication, you should make sure the doctor confirms that he or she isn't experiencing a drop-in blood pressure with standing. (Note that tamsulosin — brand name Flomax — is a popular prostate medication that also causes drops in blood pressure.)

A 2009 study of Medicare patients coming to the emergency room after fainting found that checking sitting and standing blood pressure was the most useful test. However, it was only done by doctors 1/3 of the time.
For more information, see "6 Steps to Better High Blood Pressure Treatment for Older Adults".

Don't Fall!
I'm Falling but, I'm getting up!

3. Blood tests. Checking an older person's blood tests is often a good idea after a fall. Falls can be worsened by problems with an older person's blood count, or by things like blood sodium getting too high or too low.

4. Medications review. Many older adults are taking medications that increase fall risk. These medications can often be reduced, or even eliminated. Be sure to ask the doctor to address the types of medications:

5. A physical therapist can often recommend suitable strengthening exercises, and also can help fit the older person for an assistive device (e.g. a walker) if appropriate. For more on the proven Otago physical therapy program to reduce falls — including videos demonstrating the exercises — see "Otago and Proven Exercises for Fall Prevention."

6. Vitamin D level. Studies suggest that treating low vitamin D levels (e.g. less than 20ng/mL) might help reduce falls in

Don't Fall!
I'm Falling but, I'm getting up!

older adults. Low vitamin D levels can also contribute to fragile bones.

If your older loved one spends a lot of time indoors and doesn't take a daily vitamin D supplement, there is a fairly high chance of having a low vitamin D level.

Taking a daily supplement of 800-1000 IU will eventually maintain vitamin D at a normal level in most people, but if you are very concerned about falls or vitamin D, talk to your doctor about getting a level checked. When vitamin D levels are very low, doctors sometimes treat with higher doses of vitamin D for a few months.

7. Evaluation for underlying heart conditions or neurological conditions. These chronic conditions are different from the "acute" types of illnesses that we usually look for right after a fall.

In a minority of cases, an older person may be falling because he or she has developed a chronic problem with the heart or blood pressure system. An example of this would be paroxysmal rapid atrial fibrillation, which causes the

Don't Fall!
I'm Falling but, I'm getting up!

heart to sometimes race. to the doctor about whether these services might help.

8 Things the Doctors Should Check After a Fall https://betterhealthwhileaging.net/8-things-to-check-after-fall-in-aging/.
Vision, podiatry, and home safety referrals. Could your loved one need a vision check, podiatry care, or a home safety evaluation? If you've brought an older person in after a fall, it's a good idea to talk

Seniors that fall should take specific steps that possibly reduces the risk of further injury. The first step, as hard as it likely sounds, is to not panic. Panicking potentially prevents you from accurately assessing the situation after your fall.

Do you have a medical alert system? Follow procedures and make notification right away. Medical alert systems are of great assistance when a fall occurs.
If you cannot get up, do not risk further damage or injury by attempting to force yourself to stand. If you decide to try to get up, roll to one side, and then slowly pull yourself up on all fours, until you are

Don't Fall!
I'm Falling but, I'm getting up!

on your hands and knees. If there is no sturdy object nearby, crawl to a sturdy object.

Push on the object with your hands, supporting your body weight with your hands and slowly rise to a sitting position on the steps or sturdy piece of furniture. Remain seated until confident that you can stand.

It is a good idea to always be checked out at your doctor's office or hospital emergency room when you fall, even if you think you do not have injuries. Many injuries do not exhibit symptoms right away.

Don't Fall!
I'm Falling but, I'm getting up!

Chapter 6 Risks, Causes and Reasons for Falls.

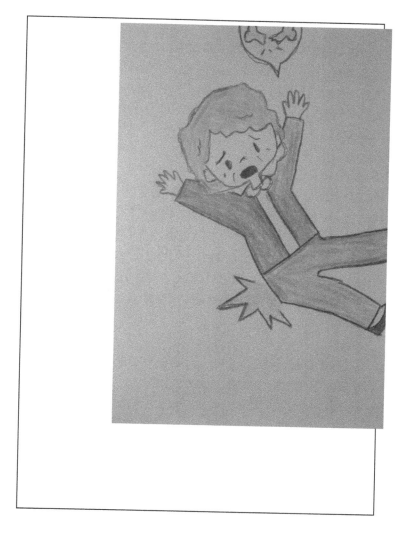

Don't Fall!
I'm Falling but, I'm getting up!

Who is at most risk for falls?
Across all age

The <u>Journal of the American Medical Association</u> published an analysis of clinical trials spanning at least a year involving participants 60 years of age and older.

Review
 Overall, the review covered 46 studies and over 20,000 participants. It concluded that rising trends of falls in the elderly statistics may be reduced by long-term exercise such as moderate aerobic, strength, and balance training.

Trial
 In the trial, the exercise frequency was three times a week for about an hour per session.

Our elderly falls statistics confirm that older people have the highest fall risk. According to a global report on falls, the risk and frequency increases with age and the deterioration of the physical condition.

Don't Fall!
I'm Falling but, I'm getting up!

Fall Rates
Fall rates are higher in elderly people living in nursing homes, and 40% of them suffer repeat falls. Additionally, women are more likely to suffer fall injuries than men, across all age groups except 75- to 79-year-olds.

How can the risk of falling be reduced? When it comes to preventing seniors' falls, the checklist for your home should first include removing any environmental hazards. Clutter or even simple home disrepair can be dangerous to elderly people living independently. In both care facilities and the home, good lighting and the use of non-slip mats are helpful. Other helpful measures include wearing clothing and shoes that fit appropriately and undergoing regular check-ups to identify and address fall-related conditions early on.

Regular exercise is another great preventative measure.

The <u>Journal of the American Medical Association</u> published an analysis of

Don't Fall!
I'm Falling but, I'm getting up!

clinical trials spanning at least a year involving participants 60 years of age and older. Overall, the review covered 46 studies and over 20,000 participants. It concluded that rising trends of falls in the elderly statistics may be reduced by long-term exercise such as moderate aerobic, strength, and balance training. In the trial, the exercise frequency was three times a week for about an hour per session.

Reasons Seniors Are at Risk of Falls
There are several reasons that contribute to the high numbers of seniors that fall. Difficulties with balance, walking and lower body weakness increase the risk of falling.

Gait and balance changes due to the aging process are not the only ways that that this issue increases the risk of falling. Certain medical conditions that affect gait and balance, such as Parkinson's disease increase the risk of falling.
Osteoporosis, the thinning of bone tissue and loss of bone density increases the risk of a fall resulting in a hip fracture.
Foot pain and wearing poorly fitting footwear also contribute to senior falls.

Don't Fall!
I'm Falling but, I'm getting up!

Other causes include Vitamin D deficiency and side effects of some prescription medications and over-the-counter medications.

Do you or a senior loved one have vision issues caused by cataracts, myopia or another issue? Falls occur more frequently among seniors with vision issues.

Disorders of the spine, including sciatica and spinal stenosis also potentially increase the risk of seniors experiencing a fall. Joint and muscle disorders increase the likelihood of falling.

There are environmental issues that contribute to falls, such as wet or uneven floors, poor lighting, unstable furniture and hazards such as throw rugs, pets and steps.

It is a good idea to always be checked out at your doctor's office or hospital emergency room when you fall, even if you think you do not have injuries. Many injuries do not exhibit symptoms right away.

Don't Fall!
I'm Falling but, I'm getting up!

What Causes Elderly People to Fall?
Decline in Physical Fitness. Many adults become less active as they get older, which exacerbates the physical effects of aging. Failure to engage in even mild exercise on a regular basis results in reduced muscle strength, decreased bone mass, loss of balance and coordination, and reduced flexibility.

Impaired Vision. Age-related eye diseases can make it difficult, if not impossible, to detect fall hazards, such as steps, puddles and thresholds. Even if a senior is in top physical condition, failing to see obstacles or changes in ground level can lead to a nasty tumble. Refusing to follow physician recommendations for treatment, including wearing eyeglasses and using necessary low vision equipment can lead to a fall as well.

Medications. A wide variety of medications can increase a senior's risk of falling. Side-effects, such as drowsiness, dizziness and low blood pressure, can all contribute to an accident. Sedatives, anti-depressants, anti-psychotics, opioids and some

Don't Fall!
I'm Falling but, I'm getting up!

cardiovascular drugs are the most common culprits.

According to the Merck Manual, just over 40 percent of seniors take at least five drugs per week. Taking multiple medications increases the risk of medication interactions and falling. Keep in mind that over-the-counter medications and supplements can have powerful side effects and synergistic effects, too.

Chronic Diseases. Health conditions such as Parkinson's disease, Alzheimer's disease and arthritis cause weakness in the extremities, poor grip strength, balance disorders and cognitive impairment. Poor physical health increases a person's initial risk of falling and minimizes their ability to respond to and recover from hazards, like tripping or slipping.

Peripheral neuropathy, or nerve damage, can cause numbness in the feet, making it very difficult for a senior to sense environmental hazards and get around safely.

Surgical Procedures.

Don't Fall!
I'm Falling but, I'm getting up!

Hip replacements and other surgeries can leave an elderly person weak, in pain and discomfort, and less mobile than they were before the procedure. This can be temporary while a patient heals or a new and lasting problem.

Environmental Hazards. The majority of falls in the elderly population occur in or around seniors' homes. Environmental factors such as poor lighting, clutter, areas of disrepair, loose carpets, slick floors and lack of safety equipment can jeopardize a senior's safety in their home. Behavioral Hazards.

A person's fall risk is influenced by their unique lifestyle and behaviors. This includes the types of activities they engage in, the level of physical demand these activities require, and their willingness and ability to adapt their routine for enhanced safety.

For example, laundry is a normal daily activity for many people, but it can involve a great deal of exertion for a senior, especially if they transport a heavy laundry basket.

Don't Fall!
I'm Falling but, I'm getting up!

This can be risky on its own, but if they also refuse to wear secure, non-skid footwear or attempt to navigate stairs, they put themselves at greater risk. Failing to modify behaviors to account for new or increasing difficulties is a serious, yet common, contributing factor for falls in older individuals.

A fall rarely occurs due to only one of the reasons above. When any of these factors combine, it can lead to a serious, possibly life-threatening injury. Even if a loved one is lucky to escape a fall uninjured, the experience can leave them shaken.

The fear of falling again can cause them to withdraw and become more sedentary, which often leads to further physical and even mental decline. To keep your loved one safe and healthy, learn how you can modify their home and lifestyle to prevent fall-related injuries.
https://www.agingcare.com/Articles/Falls-in-elderly-people-133953.htm

Don't Fall!
I'm Falling but, I'm getting up!

Chapter 7 Type of Injuries from Falls.

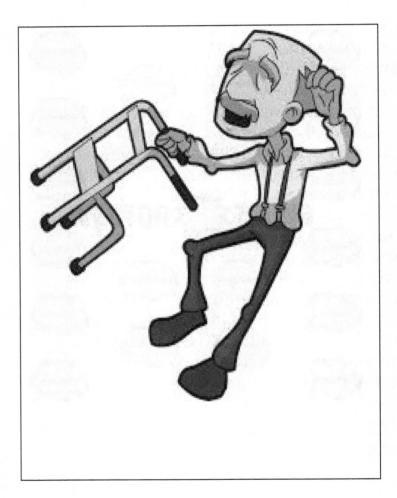

Don't Fall!
I'm Falling but, I'm getting up!

Types of Injuries from Falls
Hip Fracture, Lacerations, fractures of
spine, pelvis, legs, ankles
Men are more likely to die from a fall,
compared to a woman that experiences a
fatal fall. Medicine Net explains that in
1999, U.S.

Supreme Court Justice Harry Blackmun
died after complications from hip surgery
due to a fall at home. The fall and
subsequent death of the 90-year-old
Supreme Court Justice is just one
example of how advancing age potentially
contributes to a greater risk of serious
injury among seniors that experience a
fall.

Up to 30 percent of seniors that fall
experience a hip fracture, hip lacerations
or head trauma. In fact, falls are the most-
common cause of traumatic brain injuries
(TBI).
Falls account for the majority of all
fractures occurring in the senior
population.

Don't Fall!
I'm Falling but, I'm getting up!

Examples of these fractures, in addition to hip fractures, include fractures of the spine, pelvis, legs, ankles, upper arms, hands, and forearms upper arms, hands, and forearms. Although men have a greater risk of dying from a fall, compared to women, elderly women are more likely to experience a serious injury.

Don't Fall!
I'm Falling but, I'm getting up!

Chapter 8 After Fall.

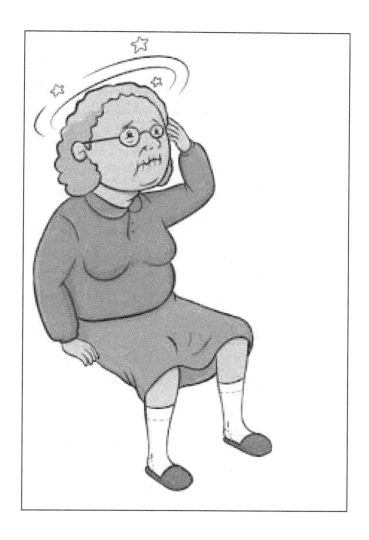

Don't Fall!
I'm Falling but, I'm getting up!

What Can Happen After a Fall?
Many falls do not cause injuries. But one out of five falls does cause a serious injury such as a broken bone or a head injury.4,5 These injuries can make it hard for a person to get around, do everyday activities, or live on their own.
Falls can cause broken bones, like wrist, arm, ankle, and hip fractures.
Falls can cause head injuries. These can be very serious, especially if the person is taking certain medicines (like blood thinners). An older person who falls and hits their head should see their doctor right away to make sure they don't have a brain injury.
Many people who fall, even if they're not injured, become afraid of falling. This fear may cause a person to cut down on their everyday activities. When a person is less active, they become weaker and this increases their chances of falling.12

Don't Fall!
I'm Falling but, I'm getting up!

Chapter 9 Injuries from Falls

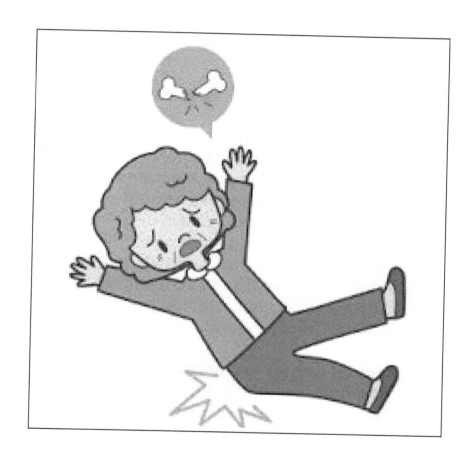

Don't Fall!
I'm Falling but, I'm getting up!

Injuries from Falls (Celebrities, Politics, Medicine, International Leaders, Religion

News reports
Injuries from a Fall
Senate Majority Leader Mitch McConnell
08/2019

On Saturday, Senate Majority Leader Mitch McConnell fell at his home in Kentucky, fracturing his shoulder.
A Saturday statement from his communications director said, "This morning, Leader McConnell tripped at home on his outside patio and suffered a fractured shoulder. He has been treated, released, and is working from home in Louisville."
Medical Center in Nashville to remove a damaged part of his lung. It was injured when he was assaulted by an angry neighbor in November 2017.

Ozzy Osbourne has now been forced to cancel all of his 2019 tour dates after falling at his home and reaggravating a 15-year-old-injury.

Don't Fall!
I'm Falling but, I'm getting up!

According to the legendary rocker, he "fell at his Los Angeles home aggravating years-old injuries (from his 2003 ATV accident) that required surgery last month."

As a result, his entire 2019 tour slate — which included North America and Europe — is canceled.

https://thelatestbreakingnews.com/ozzy-osbourne-cancels-all-2019-live-shows-after-fall-at-home/

https://globalnews.ca/news/5131021/ozzy-osbourne-postpones-tour/

Zig Ziglar In 2007, a fall down a flight of stairs left him with short-term memory problems. Nonetheless, Ziglar continued taking part in motivational seminars until he retired in 2010.[4]

Zig Ziglar's motto

Death

On November 28, 2012, Ziglar died from pneumonia at a hospital in Plano, Texas.[10]

Christina McGagh

Tim Healy

February 21, 2019 2:30 AM

Multiple rib fractures were not identified when a woman who had fallen downstairs

Don't Fall!
I'm Falling but, I'm getting up!

was X-rayed, and she died five months later, the High Court heard.
Grandmother-of-six Christina McGagh (75) had seven fractures to her ribs and was in pain when she was brought to St Luke's Hospital Carlow-Kilkenny after the fall down her stairs at home, the court was told.
The family's counsel Patrick Treacy said if she had been properly treated, it was their case that she would have fully recovered.
Ms. McGagh, from Ballon, Co Carlow, died in March 2013, five months after she fell down the stairs, counsel said.
An apology was read to the court as Ms. McGagh's son, who had sued the HSE on behalf of the family, settled his High Court action for €265,000. St Luke's and the HSE

Sources: CNN, Courier Journal

President Carter falls, breaks hip
Former president Jimmy Carter is recovering from surgery after a fall Monday morning in which he broke his hip.
The Carter Center said in a statement that Carter, 94, was leaving his home in Plains,

Don't Fall!
I'm Falling but, I'm getting up!

Ga., to go turkey hunting when he fell. The former president was recovering at Phoebe Sumter Medical Center in Americus, Ga., after surgery that his surgeon said was successful. His wife, Rosalynn, was with him.

Ed McMahon, Johnny Carson's former sidekick tripped and fell in his home on March 4, 2005. McMahon, 82 suffered from a mild concussion and a gash in his head that required stitches. He was released from the Los Angeles area hospital a few days later.

On January 19th, 2013, veteran news journalist Barbara Walters, 83, missed a step and fell on a staircase at the British Ambassador's residence in Washington D.C. prior to President Obama's second inauguration. Hospitalized to treat a cut on her forehead and subsequent low-grade fever, Walters reported that she expects to be home soon.

On May 25, 2012, musician Doc Watson, 89, fell in his home. After being taken to the hospital, it was determined he did not break any bones, but needed to undergo

Don't Fall!
I'm Falling but, I'm getting up!

colon surgery and is in critical but stable condition.

In April 2012, Kurt Masur, the eighty-four-year-old former director of the New York Philharmonic, fell off the podium into the audience while conducting in France. He was taken to the hospital where no major injuries were found.

Legendary UCLA basketball coach John Wooden fell in his condominium on Friday, February 29th, 2008, breaking his wrist and collarbone. Wooden was admitted to a local hospital and it is expected he will make a full recovery.

Beyoncé Knowles, one of the most popular singers in the world today, fell during a concert. Performing in central Florida on July 24th, 2007, Knowles tripped on her dress while trying to descend a flight of stairs. The singer fell and landed on her face, but was well enough to continue on with her routine.

On January 19th, 2013, veteran news journalist Barbara Walters, 83, missed a step and fell on a staircase at the British Ambassador's residence in Washington D.C. prior to President Obama's second

Don't Fall!
I'm Falling but, I'm getting up!

inauguration. Hospitalized to treat a cut on her forehead and subsequent low-grade fever, Walters reported that she expects to be home soon.

On May 25, 2012, musician Doc Watson, 89, fell in his home. After being taken to the hospital, it was determined he did not break any bones, but needed to undergo colon surgery and is in critical but stable condition.

In April 2012, Kurt Masur, the eighty-four-year-old former director of the New York Philharmonic, fell off the podium into the audience while conducting in France. He was taken to the hospital where no major injuries were found.

Paula Abdul is known for her bubbly but benign feedback to contestants on the hit show, American Idol. On May 22, 2007, however, the gorgeous and spunky media diva fell while trying not to step on a much smaller set of toes – those of her pet Chihuahua. While "chubby little Tulip" escaped unscathed, the forty-four-year-old former cheerleader suffered bruising from her arm to her hip, a fractured toe and a broken nose.

Musician Ryan Adams had a fall during a concert in the UK in 2004.

Don't Fall!
I'm Falling but, I'm getting up!

Tony-winning star of the Broadway musical "Wicked" Idina Menzel fell during her performance and cracked a lower rib in January 2005.
Kelsey Grammer, the star of the hit television comedy "Frasier" took a fall while on stage as the master of ceremonies at California Disneyland's 50th anniversary celebration in May 2005. Fortunately, the actor was not seriously hurt.
Nancy Reagan, the 84-year-old widow of former US president Ronald Reagan, was briefly treated in a British hospital after she fell in her hotel room in London.

In Politics
Secretary of State Hillary Clinton had another fall, this time while boarding a plane. On January 12th, 2011, the former First Lady was traveling to Yemen when she tripped and fell while walking into the plane, but was unhurt.
Former First Lady and current Secretary of State Hillary Clinton fell and broke her elbow on June 17th, 2009 while walking on her way to the White House.
Supreme Court justice Sonia Sotomayor fell and broke her ankle on

Don't Fall!
I'm Falling but, I'm getting up!

June 8th, 2009, while rushing through New York's LaGuardia airport.
Former First Lady Nancy Reagan was hospitalized after falling at her home on Sunday, February 17th. She was released after a brief, 2-night stay.
Supreme Court Chief Justice John Roberts fell while at his vacation home in Port Clyde, Maine. Chief Justice Roberts was taken to the hospital as a precautionary measure and it was later determined that the fall was caused by a seizure sustained by the Chief Justice. According to sources, Roberts fell 5 to 10 feet, which caused only minor scrapes and bruises. He is expected to stay overnight in a local hospital as a precaution.
The nation's first Commissioner on Aging died after complications from a fall. William D. Bechill was one of the nation's leading experts on Social Security, long-term care and senior centers. Mr. Bechill also played a critical role in writing the Older Americans Act, which allowed for grants supporting community service programs, research and training projects in the field of ageing.

Don't Fall!
I'm Falling but, I'm getting up!

Former Democratic presidential candidate George McGovern was hospitalized on December 2nd, 2011 after he fell and hit his head on the pavement while entering a library bearing his name, where he was set to be interviewed on C-SPAN.

In International News

Cuban President Fidel Castro tripped and fell after leaving the stage at a graduation ceremony in October 2004.

Mexican pop star Juan Gabriel suffered in a fall from a stage during a performance in Houston in 2005. Gabriel fell just minutes into the opening set of his performance at the Toyota Center and broke his wrist and suffered a concussion.

Queen Mother suffered a slight fall and cut her arm in her sitting room at Sandringham in February 2002.

In Medicine

Dr. Robert Atkins, the "weight-loss guru" that brought to us the famous "Atkins diet" died on April 17, 2003 in New York from head injuries suffered in a fall near his office. He was 72.

In Journalism

Alistair Cooke known for his BBC series "Letter from America." suffered a fall in

Don't Fall!
I'm Falling but, I'm getting up!

his Manhattan home in October 2003.
Read one journalist's farewell to "the best broadcaster on four continents."

In Religion
Pope Benedict XVI underwent surgery to repair his wrist after he fell and broke it while walking in his room on July 17th, 2009.
The Rev. Harry R. Butman, a Congregational church minister for 72 years and a prolific writer about theology and the spiritual life, has passed away. He was 101.Butman died in 2005 at his home in Acton of complications from a fall.
Marj Carpenter, the ex-director of the Presbyterian News Service fell and suffered a broken hip in November 2000 while trying to enter a car outside her home in Texas.
Billy Graham, the popular evangelist who is now 86 years old, suffered from two falls in 2004 that resulted in fractures. After his recuperation, he has been able to continue traveling and preaching in various cities.
Benjamin Goodman Karim, 73, a minister and author and a right-hand man to Malcolm X during the civil rights

Don't Fall!
I'm Falling but, I'm getting up!

movement, died Aug. 2 of 2005 after a fall
in Richmond, where he resided.
Those Who Have Fallen in the Past
John Herschel Glenn Jr., former American
pilot, astronaut, and politician.
"Glenn had originally planned to enter
politics earlier, but in 1966 had suffered a
fall in his bathtub, sustaining a concussion
as well as injuring his inner ear, and
recovery left him unable to campaign at
that time." Click here for more about Mr.
John H. Glenn Jr.
Famous Faller: Hillary Clinton
Famous Faller: Pope Benedict XVI
Pope Benedict XVI breaks wrist in
bathroom fall while on holiday
Pope Benedict XVI will spend the next
month with his wrist in a cast after he
broke it when he slipped over in the
bathroom of a holiday chalet.

By Nick Pisa in Perugia
2:48PM BST 17 Jul 2009
The 82-year-old Pontiff, who was enjoying
a two-week summer break in the Italian
Alps, tripped over during the night as he
was leaving a bathroom next to his
bedroom. He twists his ankle and
fractured his right wrist.

Don't Fall!
I'm Falling but, I'm getting up!

https://www.telegraph.co.uk/news/worldnews/europe/italy/5851029/Pope-Benedict-XVI-breaks-wrist-in-bathroom-fall-while-on-holiday.html

http://stopfalls.org/what-is-fall-prevention/famous-fallers/
Barbara Bush, "the Matriarch"
April 15, 2018, her family released a statement regarding her failing health stating that she had chosen to be at home with family, desiring "comfort care" rather than further medical treatment.
According to family spokesman Jim McGrath, her decision came as a result of "a series of recent hospitalizations". Bush died in her Houston home at the age of 92 on April 17, 2018.[
Reports are alleged she fell and injured herself-was taken to hospital but never recovered (told by Author, The Matriarch, Barbara Bush Susan Page) Martha the Story, 04/2/19

Don't Fall!
I'm Falling but, I'm getting up!

Chapter 10 News reports on Deaths

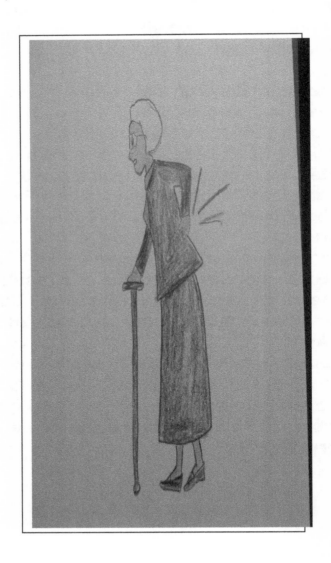

Don't Fall!
I'm Falling but, I'm getting up!

Deaths after a Fall

Wife of Oral Roberts dies after a fall Staff Reports May 5, 2005

Evelyn Roberts' death came a day after she fell in the parking lot of a dentist's office, striking her head on the pavement and causing massive internal bleeding. Taken to a nearby hospital, she lapsed into a coma and never regained consciousness.

https://www.tulsaworld.com/archive/wife-of-oral-roberts-dies-after-a-fall/article_b27fcd93-3ebd-5151-b51b-04996553ba7b.html

Supreme Court Justice Dies After Breaking Hip in Fall Reviewed on 6/13/2018
Privacy & Trust Info
On March 4, 1999 Justice Harry A. Blackmun died of complications after hip replacement surgery. He underwent the procedure after a fall at his home. Justice Blackmun was 90. The cause of Justice Blackmun's death underscores the seriousness of the consequences of a fall in the elderly and the need to understand

Don't Fall!
I'm Falling but, I'm getting up!

why such falls occur and precautions to prevent falls whenever possible.

In the Arts and Entertainment
Ann B. Davis, who played Alice the housekeeper on the popular 1960s sitcom The Brady Bunch, died on Sunday in San Antonio after entering into a coma sustained by a <u>fall in her bathtub</u>. She was 88 years old.
Actor Robert Culp, best known for his role in the hit 1960s TV show, "I Spy", died on March 24th, 2010.
Dave Freeman, whose book "100 Things To Do Before You Die" inspired the recent film "The Bucket List", died after <u>hitting his head from a fall at his home</u>. He was 47.
Famed country singer Eddy Arnold, who's career included 28 No. 1 records, broke his hip when he <u>fell at his Brentwood, KY home</u>. He recently <u>passed away</u> while at a Nashville, TN area care facility.
<u>Frank Butler OBE</u>, 89, one of Britain's best-known sports writers, passed away in hospital on Jan 29th of 2006 following a fall at his home in Chislehurst, Kent. He was a sports editor of the News of the World for 25 years and retired 23 years

Don't Fall!
I'm Falling but, I'm getting up!

ago. He covered boxing from the era of Joe Louis, was a former chairman of the Boxing Writers Club and former steward of the British Boxing Board of Control. British jazz piano icon Mr. George Shearing was admitted to a New York City hospital after a fall in his home in March 2004.

Consuelo Velazquez, composer of the sustaining 1940s-era hit "BE same Macho" suffered a fall at home in Mexico City in November 2004 that left her in intensive care. She recently passed away at age 88.
Falls Death rates projected

Projection: (Falls) Death Rates
According to
www.cdc.gov/homeandRecreationalSafety
See Fall Death Rates in the US increased 30% from 2007 to 2016 for older Adults
If rates continue to rise, we can anticipate 7 Fall Deaths every Hour By 2030
www.cdc.gov
After tripping or stumbling, a younger adult can rely on strong muscles and sharp reflexes to quickly regain balance

Don't Fall!
I'm Falling but, I'm getting up!

or heal quickly from injury. But an older adult has a weaker body response and is far more likely to fall and have lasting damage – even if they're already using a walker or cane.

In fact, the <u>CDC</u> says that people age 65+ have a greater than 25% chance of falling. And if someone falls once, their chance of falling again doubles, meaning there's over 50% chance of a second fall.
This is serious because falls are a leading cause of lost independence and ability.

<u>Seniors</u> often aren't able to recover fully from the trauma, their overall health declines, and their care needs increase significantly.
We explain the top 6 age-related changes that increase senior fall risk, typical injuries, and ways to reduce fall risk.

 1. Decreasing strength
Muscle loss starts very early, around age 30. In older adults, less muscle means less strength and weaker bones.

2. Weaker sense of balance
Many body systems work together to keep

Don't Fall!
I'm Falling but, I'm getting up!

us standing upright. Age-related changes and medication side effects can make it more difficult for seniors to stay balanced.

3. Declining eyesight
Vision helps us keep our balance and avoid obstacles. As vision worsens, so does the ability to stay upright and clearly see what's in our path.

4. Loss of flexibility
Age and health conditions make seniors less flexible, especially in hips and ankles. This stiffness increases the likelihood of falling.

5. Decreased endurance
Not being able to endure physical activity like standing or walking for a reasonable amount of time will increase fall risk.

6. Declining ability and desire to walk
Continuing to walk will improve strength, balance, flexibility, and endurance for older adults.
https://dailycaring.com/why-do-seniors-fall-down/

Don't Fall!
I'm Falling but, I'm getting up!

However, many seniors become less active and fall into a negative cycle where less activity leads to less strength and balance. That leads to even less activity as their physical abilities keep declining.

CDC: Falls-Related Deaths in the US Rose 31% in 10 Years, May 2018

Among US residents age 65 and older, the rate of death from falls continues to climb steadily, having increased by 31% between 2007 and 2016, and growing at a particularly rapid rate among those aged 85 and above.

The latest statistics, included in a report from the US Centers for Disease Control and Prevention (CDC), point to a need for more widespread falls screening and prevention efforts including physical therapy, authors say.

During the 10 years tracked in the study, falls-related deaths among US residents 65 and older rose from 18,334 to 29,668—in terms of rates of death from falls, that's an increase from 47 per 100,000 to 61.6 per 100,000 in that age group. Deaths

Don't Fall!
I'm Falling but, I'm getting up!

climbed by about 3% per year, according to the report.
In addition to overall totals and rates, CDC researchers looked at data in terms of demographics and state-by-state variables.

Among their findings:
In 2016, falls-related deaths per 100,000 were highest among white non-Hispanic US residents (68.7) and the all-ethnicity 85-and-older group (257.9).

While death rates increased for all age groups, the 85-and-older category recorded the most dramatic rise between 2007 and 2016, from 9,188 deaths in 2007 to 16,454 in 2016. The 65-to-74 age group recorded 2,594 falls-related deaths in 2007 and 4,479 in 2016; the 75-to-84 age group saw an increase from 6,552 deaths in 2007 to 8,735 in 2016.

Men had higher rates of falls-related deaths than did women—73.2 per 100,000 men compared with 54 per 100,000 per women. Researchers believe the gap may be attributable to "differences in the circumstances of a fall," with men tending

Don't Fall!
I'm Falling but, I'm getting up!

to experience falls that lead to more serious injuries, such as those sustained in a fall from a ladder or as the result of alcohol consumption.

Rates for deaths from falls in the 65-and-older age group varied among states, ranging from 142.7 per 100,000 in Wisconsin to 24.4 per 100,000 in Alabama.

Authors aren't sure of the reasons for the variance but suspect that the numbers might be related to demographic variables including differing proportions of older white adults in various states.

Another possible explanation cited in the report was the impact of who completes the death certificate: According to the CDC researchers, a 2012 study showed that coroners reported 14% fewer deaths from falls than did medical examiners.

Authors of the report theorize that the rates of falls-related deaths may be climbing in part because of an aging population and longer survival rates after common diseases including heart disease, cancer, and stroke.

Don't Fall!
I'm Falling but, I'm getting up!

Whatever the contributing factors, it's a trend that needs to be addressed, they write: even if the rate were to stabilize, an estimated 43,000 US residents would die from falls in 2030, and if the rate were to climb as it did from 2007 to 2016, some 59,000 individuals may die from falls in 2030.
"As the US population aged [65 and older] increases,
Caution: You're entering the "No Fall" Zone

Don't Fall!
I'm Falling but, I'm getting up!

Chapter 11 Fall Prevention Exercise and Activities.

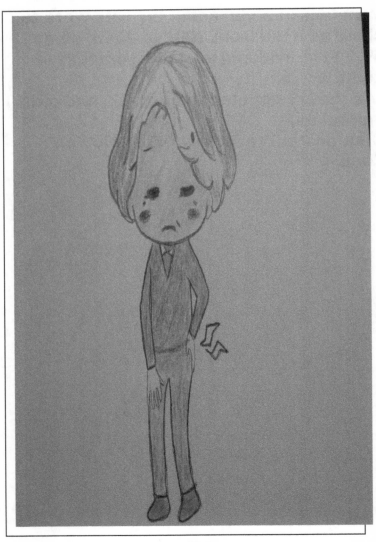

Don't Fall!
I'm Falling but, I'm getting up!

How to Stop Falling
Prevention is key

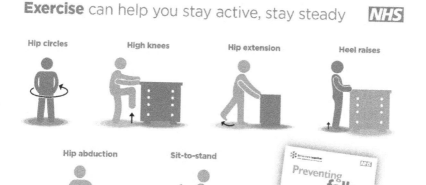

15 Ways to Reduce Fall Risk and Help Prevent Falls
Begin with the bathroom. Wet surfaces (on the floor or counters) can be very dangerous. Seniors lack the balance and reaction time needed to avoid a fall. While it may seem easy to step out of a shower, an unsteady senior may slip and come crashing to the floor. To help, provide

Don't Fall!
I'm Falling but, I'm getting up!

non-slip mats in the bathtub and shower. Install grab bars in strategic points around the bathroom. Towel bars are not sufficient because they will collapse under someone's full body weight. Grab bars can be attached inside the shower stall or just above the bathtub to help a senior with lowering or standing up. Provide a shower seat. Seniors can be far more secure when they are seated when showering.

Replace the shower head with a hand-held nozzle. Seniors can become more confident with showering with a nozzle. The nozzle can be easily turned away in the case of sudden water temperature changes. In addition, it can result in a much more thorough cleaning. Long-hoses are now available, which are far easier to use for someone seated in the shower.

Stairs. Whether inside or outside the senior's home, stairs can be major concerns. I recall my parent's first retirement home in Victoria, British Columbia. This was a beautiful two-bedroom condo with a view of the ocean

Don't Fall!
I'm Falling but, I'm getting up!

but outside access proved to be too much. I often saw my mother grabbing the handrail and pulling herself up the stairs to get inside. If a senior does have stairs, there are plenty of precautions you can take.

Clear the stairs. Whether it is a few dropped clothes or a grandchild's toy, anything left on the stairs can become a tripping and falling hazard.

Differentiate between the stairs. Aging eyes may not always be able to separate one step from the next. To help, you could try replacing the carpet on each step to make the steps easier to spot. In the case of bare steps, try painting each step a different color. Other options include adding safety tape or removing carpeting and adding stair treads. All flights of stairs should also have handrails on both sides of the stairs.

Consider a stairlift. These mechanisms can safely take a senior up or down a flight of stairs. The senior will sit in a comfortable chair without having to climb up or down the stairs. A colleague of mine

Don't Fall!
I'm Falling but, I'm getting up!

used this with her father. This enabled her and her family to turn the basement into a fully furnished suite for him and his caregiver.

Shovel snow and chip ice off stairs in the winter. This work can be too much for a senior to handle. So why not delegate the job to a younger family caregiver or hire a neighbor? This task prevents slipping and falling outside the home.

Tighten stair handrails. A loose handrail is of little good to anyone grabbing for it. Secure these handrails both inside and outside the senior's home.

Tuck away extension cords. Are there any power cords stretched across a senior's floor? Tape them down or slide them underneath or behind furniture.

Remove excess furniture. A more mobile senior may be able to sidestep a footstool or a coffee table but not all seniors can do this. Remove unneeded furniture to give the senior more room to maneuver and help to create a safer living environment. Also, a deep plush armchair may look

Don't Fall!
I'm Falling but, I'm getting up!

comfortable, but the senior may become trapped if he or she lacks the body strength necessary to push up and out of the chair.

Get a cane or a walker. A doctor can best advise if the senior will need a mobility aid. This could be a wheelchair, a walker, a cane, or a motorized scooter. As with any mobility aid, make sure that is properly fitted for the best and easiest use. Reducing or eliminating the walker stigma that often exists may be a little more difficult to do. However, seniors may find that using a walker increases their own freedom, independence, and quality of life. Be aware that an occupational therapist needs to train the person to use these properly.

For increased convenience, choose a wheelchair, walker, or scooter that can collapse and fit easily in a car's trunk or back seat. Be mindful of the size of mobility aids. A wheelchair or walker may be too wide to fit through a senior's doorways. A four-wheeled scooter will be better for outdoor use and will provide more stability. A three-wheeled scooter

Don't Fall!
I'm Falling but, I'm getting up!

can be far more maneuverable inside the home.
Evaluate a senior's footwear. Shoes need to fit well and have non-slip soles. Shoes with Velcro straps can be easier to tighten or loosen. They also remove any risk of tripping over long laces. Do not choose senior's shoes based on how easily they can be put on and taken off. I've heard from at least one person whose father wore loose shoes and she had to buy all new shoes for him.

Install better, brighter lighting. Seniors cannot always see that well in a dark or shadowed room. Better, brighter lighting can help to light the way. On this same subject, assess the location of light switches. These may be out of reach for someone in a wheelchair.

Keep a senior active. Whether through regular walking or light exercising and stretching, an active senior can remain more stable than a sedentary senior. Exercising can help prevent falls by keeping stabilizing muscles strong.
https://homecareassistance.com/blog/4-

Don't Fall!
I'm Falling but, I'm getting up!

<u>long-term-consequences-of-falls-among-older-adults</u>

Seniors engage in certain prevention exercises and activities; they likely decrease their risk of falling. Increasing strength, flexibility, and balance likely helps seniors improve stability and walking.

Consider Tai Chi or yoga, popular activities that do not require difficult, painful movements that sometimes lead to seniors avoiding regular exercise. Enjoy bicycling and reduce your risk of falling while increasing the strength in your legs.

While seniors often fear falling, failing to engage in regular exercise and activities potentially results in further physical decline, social isolation, feelings of helplessness and depression among seniors, explains the National Council on Aging.

<u>Exercise</u>
The most effective single intervention is exercise. Exercises that improve lower body strength, balance, and coordination

Don't Fall!
I'm Falling but, I'm getting up!

are the most helpful, and these can be done as group classes or individual at-home programs

Management Medication: Physicians and pharmacists should review all the medications that are being taken, even over-the-counter medicines. As individuals get older, the way medicines work in the body can change. Some medications, or combinations of medications, can make individuals sleepy and dizzy, at times.

Know More Prevention Tips
Learning some fall prevention tips for the elderly is necessary in keeping them safe. Upon reaching your senior years, it is crucial to start researching. Here is a fall prevention checklist with techniques that can be implemented at home.

1. Move
Regular physical activity is vital for seniors. Even if you are just at home, make sure to allow your body to move regularly. Gentle fall prevention exercises include walking, tai chi, water workouts and graceful and slow dance-like

Don't Fall!
I'm Falling but, I'm getting up!

movements (more examples). This helps in reducing your risk of experiencing falls because these promote improved strength, flexibility, coordination and balance.
For physically stronger seniors, swimming is a good exercise to consider. According to a 2014 study, Swimming Can Help To Prevent Senior Falls.

2. Fall-Proof Your Home
Fall-proofing your home involves removing safety hazards from it. Improving or adding sufficient lighting is also necessary in preventing seniors from falling because of difficulty seeing objects. Installing grab bars and handrails and arranging items at home and storing them in a place where you can easily reach them is also beneficial. Strategically placing specially designed fall mats in places where falls are likely to occur offers protection should falls unfortunately happen.

3. Remove Clutter
Make your home as clutter-free as possible by removing unnecessary furniture and other unused objects. The

Don't Fall!
I'm Falling but, I'm getting up!

furniture items that remain in your home should also be stable. Make sure that these are devoid of sharp corners to minimize injuries in case of accidental trips.

4. Use the Right Footwear
Wear a pair of shoes that properly fit and comes with non-skid holes. Stay away from high heels. It is also vital to tie your shoelaces. Another tip is to avoid walking in your stocking feet and wearing slippers that have already gone too loose or stretched out of their regular shape.

5. Maintain an Organized Kitchen
Effective fall prevention also involves organizing all the items in your kitchen. Removing throw rugs and cleaning up all liquids, food and grease spilled over your kitchen floor is also a must. Storing items for cooking and consumption such as food ingredients, cooking equipment and dishes in an easy to reach area is also helpful.

Don't Fall!
I'm Falling but, I'm getting up!

6. Improve the Safety of Your Bathroom
Use a slip-resistant rug in your bathroom and install grab bars into the wall. Make sure the bathroom has sufficient lighting when used. Adding a nightlight into your bathroom can also help.
Replacing shower enclosures made of glass with non-shattering material can also reduce your risk of falling. Using a raised or special toilet seat featuring armrests can also help in enhancing your stability in the toilet.

7. Visit your Eye Doctor
Remember that poor vision or eyesight is one of the leading causes of falling in the elderly. This means that fall prevention in the elderly involves getting vision problems corrected. Visit your eye doctor regularly and use up to date prescription lens.

8. Manage Your Medications
Ask your pharmacist or doctor to review all the over the counter and prescription medications you are taking. This is helpful in identifying which ones trigger side effects like drowsiness and dizziness that often lead to falls.

Don't Fall!
I'm Falling but, I'm getting up!

9. Take Advantage of Devices Designed to Aid the Elderly
These include handrails installed on the stairways, raised toilet seat, non-slip treads, grab bars installed in your tub or shower, and durable plastic seat for your tub or shower. Invest in these devices to make the process of moving easy for the elderly.

10. Make Sure that Your Bedroom is Well-Lit
This is one of the most important fall preventions in the home tips. Avoid getting up in the dark. A wise tip is to keep your light switch near your bed, so you can easily reach for it in case you want to get up at night. Hiding all loose extension cords in your bedroom is also beneficial in decreasing the risk of tripping over them.
http://medicalalertsystemshq.com/fall-prevention/10-fall-prevention-tips-for-the-elderly.html

Risk Assessments
Seniors can take a number of precautions to prevent falls. Reminders

Don't Fall!
I'm Falling but, I'm getting up!

Exercise regularly. <u>Do exercises</u> that will increase leg strength, improve balance and increase flexibility. Consider Tai Chi, <u>yoga</u>, and bicycling.
Review your medications with your doctor or pharmacist. You'll want to reduce or eliminate those that cause dizziness or drowsiness.

Lower your hip fracture risk by getting daily-recommended levels of calcium and vitamin D. and get screened and treated for osteoporosis.
Move furniture that's in your way. Use double-sided tape so throw rugs won't slip.

Pick up items that are on the floor. Coil telephone and electrical wires next to the wall.
Keep items off the stairs. Fix loose or uneven steps.
Make sure your stairway is lighted and have switches at the top and bottom of the stairs.
Make sure stair carpeting is secure.
Make sure stair handrails are secure and that they're on both sides the entire length of the stairs.

Don't Fall!
I'm Falling but, I'm getting up!

Consider a walk-in tub to ensure easy entrance and exit.
When using a ladder, make sure both feet and at least one hand are on the ladder.
Consider buying an alarm you can activate in the event of a fall.
Get up slowly when lying down or sitting, making sure that your path is free from clutter and obstacles.

Make sure items in the kitchen are within reach. Do you use a step stool in the kitchen? Make sure it is stable before each use.
Place a non-slip mat or strips inside your shower or bathtub to help prevent falls. Installing grab bars further decreases the risk of falling.
Use a night light in your bedroom. Make sure there is enough light for you to see inside the bedroom and along the way to the bathroom and kitchen.

Do you have throw rugs or loose carpeting? Secure the loose carpeting and use double-sided tape on rugs so that they do not slip.
See an optometrist or ophthalmologist at least annually to make sure that you do

Don't Fall!
I'm Falling but, I'm getting up!

not have vision issues that increase your risk of falling.

Elderly Fall Prevention Checklist
Learning some fall prevention tips for the elderly is necessary in keeping them safe. Upon reaching your senior years, it is crucial to start researching. Here is a fall prevention checklist with techniques that can be implemented at home.

Injury Prevention
Falls, the leading cause of injury among older adults, are treated in emergency departments every 13 seconds and claim a life every 20 minutes. Every year, 1 out of 3 older adults fall, yet less than half tell their doctor.[8] Falls-related injuries and deaths can be prevented by addressing risk factors. The Administration for Community Living supports evidence-based falls prevention programs that are implemented in community settings through aging services and other community providers. Center for Disease Control and Prevention's Stopping Elderly Accidents, Deaths, & Injuries (STEADI) tools and educational materials can assist health

Don't Fall!
I'm Falling but, I'm getting up!

care providers in reducing their patients'
risk of falling.10
The National Institute on Aging (NIA) and
the Patient-Centered Outcomes Research
Institute (PCORI) are testing evidence-
based interventions that deploy nurses or
nurse practitioners as "falls care
managers."
How can falls be
prevented?
National Institute on Aging Help people
with Alzheimer's prevent falls

As Alzheimer's disease gets worse,
the person may have trouble walking
and keeping his or her balance. He or
she also may have changes in depth
perception, which is the ability to
understand distances. For example,
someone with Alzheimer's may try to
step down when walking from a
carpeted to a tile floor. This puts him
or her at risk for falls.

To reduce the chance of a fall:
Clean up clutter.
Remove throw rugs.
Use chairs with arms.
Put grab bars in the bathroom.

Don't Fall!
I'm Falling but, I'm getting up!

Use good lighting.
Make sure the person wears sturdy
shoes with good traction.
.
https://www.nia.nih.gov/health/preven
t-falls-and-fractures

Don't Fall!
I'm Falling but, I'm getting up!

These precautions can help minimize the risk of falls:
Physical activity to improve strength, mobility, and flexibility in seniors;
Limiting <u>sleep</u>-inducing medications whenever possible;
Appropriate treatment of underlying medical conditions;
Environmental modifications such as installing grab bars, removing tripping obstacles (especially animals and rugs), and maintaining sufficient lighting;
And some common sense doesn't hurt!
This article is based in part on information from the Division of Unintentional Injury <u>Prevention</u> of the National Center for Injury Prevention and Control

Don't Fall!
I'm Falling but, I'm getting up!

Chapter 12   Medical Alert Devices Benefits.

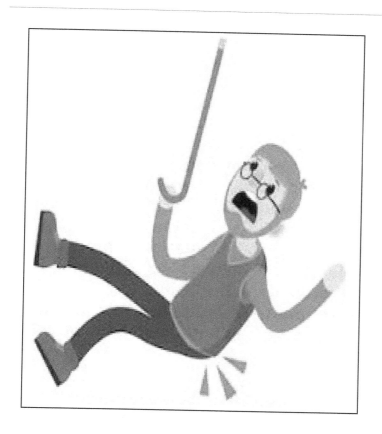

Don't Fall!
I'm Falling but, I'm getting up!

Medical alert devices potentially offer considerable benefits and reassurance when a senior fall or is at risk of falling.

AARP
The AARP revealed one incident where a woman received a call from the medical alert company operator as she made breakfast one morning. She had not heard her husband calling her from upstairs after a fall and pushed his emergency alert pendant. The woman rushed upstairs and discovered her husband bleeding profusely after hitting his head on the doorframe of the bedroom door.
This example highlights the considerable benefits of having a medical alert device.

Leah Bellman, M.S., occupational therapist and stroke rehabilitation specialist stated in a Consumer Reports article that anyone at risk of experiencing a fall or experiencing another type of medical emergency might benefit from having a medical alert device.
There are several types of medical alert devices, including the pendant style, and

Don't Fall!
I'm Falling but, I'm getting up!

speakerphone medical alert systems.
Other medical alert systems include
cellular medical alert systems,
phone/medical alert combination and the
activity tracker.

'Medical Alert Systems for Seniors.'
How do you know which medical alert
system is the best option? Deciding on the
ideal medical alert system depends on
several factors, including the variety of
features, service options and costs that
make a particular system the right choice
for your needs.

Smartphone is not enough
One important fact to note is that many
experts agree that simply relying on a
Smartphone is not enough. Most seniors
do not have their phone with them at all
times, leaving open the possibility of
falling and not having the phone with
them.

Decide whether you want a system that
operates strictly with your landline
telephone or prefer mobile medical alert
devices.

Don't Fall!
I'm Falling but, I'm getting up!

Fall Detection
The system you choose needs to have a fall detection or prevention feature, probably the most common reason that seniors choose a medical alert system.

Push Button
Make sure you choose a device that allows you to push a button to call for help, which connects you to either a live operator or emergency services such as police or medics.

GPS
GPS monitoring and location tracking is important for active seniors that drive or that enjoy walking or hiking and risk a fall.

Waterproof
Check how waterproof a medical alert system is before purchasing the system. You want to be able to wear it in the shower or bathtub.

Medical monitoring and activity monitoring
Medical monitoring and activity monitoring are additional features that

Don't Fall!
I'm Falling but, I'm getting up!

make a medical alert device an ideal option for seniors at risk of falling.

Costs
Costs of medical alert devices vary. Make sure the company you purchase a medical alert device from has no hidden fees, or complicated pricing plans. Never fall for an offer of purchasing used medical alert device equipment.

Increased Risk of Falling
Seniors are at an increased risk of falling, compared to younger people. Medical alert devices help seniors have more confidence, with many companies offering outstanding fall prevention and detection features, monitoring and excellent customer services.

Senior Fall Prevention-Serious Topic
Senior fall prevention should be a serious topic for seniors and those with seniors in their lives. The statistics show that the problem is real, and it can be serious. Fortunately, you can mitigate the risks with some preventative measures at home and exercise to strengthen your balance. Materials for Your Older Patients

Don't Fall!
I'm Falling but, I'm getting up!

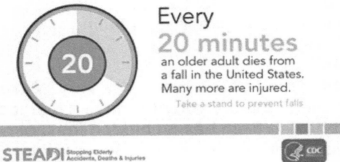

Every
20 minutes
an older adult dies from
a fall in the United States.
Many more are injured.

Take a stand to prevent falls

STEADI Stopping Elderly
Accidents, Deaths & Injuries

Falls affect us all—whether personally or someone we love or care about. Every second of every day an older adult fall. In 2015 alone, more than one in four older adults reported falling and more than 28,000 older adults died as a result of falls—that's 74 older adults every day. There are simple steps you can take to prevent falls and decrease falls risks. CDC developed the STEADI (Stopping Elderly Accidents, Deaths & Injuries) initiative which includes educational materials and tools to improve fall prevention.

What Is Fall Detection and How Does It Work?
The fall detection device can come in the form of a necklace pendant or a watch-like wristband and when triggered, can

Don't Fall!
I'm Falling but, I'm getting up!

contact a live agent or family member. Some medical alert companies like Medical Guardian include fall detection in all plans, while other medical alert providers may charge extra.
How Does it Work?

Fall detection technology is actually pretty simple. The detection device has a built-in accelerometer that constantly track the movements of the wearer. Since a fall is a sudden movement, the accelerometer picks it up instantly, processes it and makes the alert call.

Though sometimes there can be false alarms, the medical alert representative will be able to contact the wearer and determine the best <u>course of action</u>.

Features
• Waterproof – This is extremely important, considering that many old people are prone to falling in the bathroom or shower.

• Size – A fall detection device should be comfortable to wear. If it's too bulky, it won't do.

Don't Fall!
I'm Falling but, I'm getting up!

• <u>Manual</u> and Automatic Detection – Many devices today have a "Cancel" button. Therefore, if the detection is false, the wearer can let the agents know there's no problem. Moreover, if the automatic detection fails, for some reason or another, the device should have a button for a manual call.

• Ease of Use – If the detection device is too complicated, this can pose a problem for the elderly individual. Always opt for the simplest – yet most efficient – fall detection devices out there.

The Bottom Line
Fall detection devices help make sure that elderly loved ones are kept safe and can notify you in the blink of an eye if they fall.

To discover the best fall detection devices, <u>check</u> out our expert medical alert reviews Joe Schwartz
Medical Alerts Editor

Medical Alert Devices
 Download Free 2019 Medical Alert
Systems Buyer's Guide

Don't Fall!
I'm Falling but, I'm getting up!

7th Annual – Most Trusted Buying Guide in Industry

https://www.inhomesafetyguide.org/medical-guardian-rating-review/

Medical alert devices potentially offer considerable benefits and reassurance when a senior fall or is at risk of falling. Illustration: The AARP revealed one incident where a woman received a call from the medical alert company operator as she made breakfast one morning. She had not heard her husband calling her from upstairs after a fall and pushed his emergency alert pendant. The woman rushed upstairs and discovered her husband bleeding profusely after hitting his head on the doorframe of the bedroom door.

This example highlights the considerable benefits of having a medical alert device. Leah Bellman, M.S., occupational therapist and stroke rehabilitation specialist stated in a Consumer Reports article that anyone at risk of experiencing a fall or experiencing another type of medical emergency might

Don't Fall!
I'm Falling but, I'm getting up!

benefit from having a medical alert
device.
There are several types of medical alert
devices, including the pendant style, and
speakerphone medical alert systems.
Other medical alert systems include
cellular medical alert systems,
phone/medical alert combination and the
activity tracker.

How do you know which medical alert
system is the best option? Deciding on the
ideal medical alert system depends on
several factors, including the variety of
features, service options and costs that
make a particular system the right choice
for your needs.

Smartphone not enough:
One important fact to note is that many
experts agree that simply relying on a
Smartphone is not enough. Most seniors
do not have their phone with them at all
times, leaving open the possibility of
falling and not having the phone with
them.

Decide whether you want a system that
operates strictly with your landline

Don't Fall!
I'm Falling but, I'm getting up!

telephone or prefer mobile medical alert devices.
The system you choose needs to have a fall detection or prevention feature, probably the most common reason that seniors choose a medical alert system.

Make sure you choose a device that allows you to push a button to call for help, which connects you to either a live operator or emergency services such as police or medics.

GPS monitoring and location tracking is important for active seniors that drive or that enjoy walking or hiking and risk a fall. Check how waterproof a medical alert system is before purchasing the system. You want to be able to wear it in the shower or bathtub.
Medical monitoring and activity monitoring are additional features that make a medical alert device an ideal option for seniors at risk of falling.
Costs of medical alert devices vary. Make sure the company you purchase a medical alert device from has no hidden fees, or complicated pricing plans. Never fall for

Don't Fall!
I'm Falling but, I'm getting up!

an offer of purchasing used medical alert device equipment.
Seniors are at an increased risk of falling, compared to younger people. Medical alert devices help seniors have more confidence, with many companies offering outstanding fall prevention and detection features, monitoring and excellent customer services.

Don't Fall!
I'm Falling but, I'm getting up!

Chapter 13 Most Commonly Asked
Questions About Medical Alert systems.

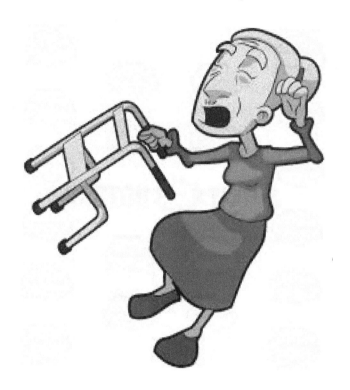

Don't Fall!
I'm Falling but, I'm getting up!

Questions & Answers

Medical alert systems bring peace of mind to <u>seniors</u> and people of all ages who live alone and have medical conditions which may require emergency assistance. Not sure which medical alert system is right for you? Find the answers to the most important questions about medical alert systems below to get started.

Who is the medical alert monitoring service right for?
Medical alert systems make sense for seniors and people of all ages that live alone or spend long periods of time alone and may require emergency <u>medical assistance</u>. This can include those with medical conditions such as epilepsy, stroke, seizures, heart conditions, or those with a likelihood to suffer from a fall. In the event of an emergency situation, the person can quickly contact operators to have them dispatch police, ambulance, or firefighters or alert designated caregivers and contacts.

What kind of services do medical alert systems provide?

Don't Fall!
I'm Falling but, I'm getting up!

In the event of a medical emergency, personal alert systems allow the user to quickly get in touch with someone to send help. The medical alert operator will be prepared with all the important contacts including family, friends, physician, etc. for effective and fast assistance in the event of an emergency. The operators can also dispatch emergency professionals such as the police, paramedics, or firefighters when necessary.

What kind of devices do medical alert systems include?
Medical alert solutions will offer a range of different devices that allow the user to instantly get help in case of a medical emergency. Medical alert systems offer different types of devices for at home or on-the-go mobile alerts.
The device may operate by pushing a button in order to communicate with an operator. At home systems usually connect to a landline, but do not require one. For more active users, the mobile alert systems provide GPS enabled systems with unlimited range. Services

Don't Fall!
I'm Falling but, I'm getting up!

may also include fall detection and other add-ons.

What are medical alert bracelets?
When it comes to medical alert equipment, carrying around a large device just isn't a practical solution. For this reason, companies have created wearable devices that users can <u>access</u> at all times. Items like medical alert bracelets allow someone to wear their alert system comfortable and conveniently around their wrist. In this way, they can bring the device anywhere they go and have full protection on-the-go. Many of these medical alert bracelets also have a fall detection feature that automatically sends an alert in the event of a fall. Fall detection could prove crucial especially if the person becomes unconscious after falling. Some medical alert systems may charge an extra fee for fall detection, but others like <u>Medical Guardian</u> have fall detection included.
Medical Alerts Editor Source: Joe Schwartz | Medical Alerts Editor
Our chief content editor, Joe manages a diverse team of content writers. He holds a degree in online communications and

Don't Fall!
I'm Falling but, I'm getting up!

his writing has been featured in a wide range of online publications. https://www.thetop10sites.com/medical-alerts/blog/benefits-of-medical-alert-systems.html

Don't Fall!
I'm Falling but, I'm getting up!

Chapter 14 Medical Alert Systems.

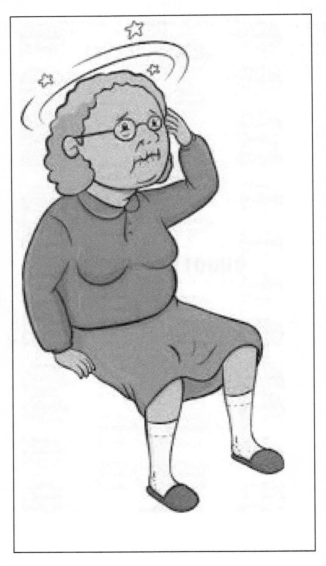

Don't Fall!
I'm Falling but, I'm getting up!

Medical Alert Systems-provides affordable alternative safety and independence

As our loved ones get older, they can become more susceptible to accidents and injuries. Spending money on a caregiver or a nursing home can incur major costs and cause a major inconvenience. Medical alert systems provide an affordable alternative to ensure a person's safety and independence.

1. Allows the Person to Remain Independent
Medical alert systems have both at-home and portable options so that both you and your family member can remain independent and maintain privacy. Your loved one won't need to be accompanied every time they leave the house.

2. Affordable
Medical alert systems like <u>Medical Guardian</u> or <u>Life Station</u> offer an affordable option for under $30 per month, while still providing crucial help around the clock. Not everyone can

Don't Fall!
I'm Falling but, I'm getting up!

afford to pay for a personal caregiver or relocating to a nursing home.

3. Avoid the Nursing Home
In addition to their high costs, <u>nursing homes</u> can be a major upheaval and interruption in a person's life. Many elderly people are comfortable in their homes and communities and moving to an unfamiliar location can be disrupting. Medical alert systems help avoid the cost and the hassle of having to relocate a loved one from their home.

4. Provides Services Cell Phones in an emergency, you can't always rely on a cell phone to call for help. Cell reception can sometimes be spotty, and cellphones are not durable and waterproof. Wearable medical alert devices ensure that the person always has the alert button with them , even in the shower. Plus, cell phones aren't always user-friendly, and involve pushing more than just one button.

5. On the Go and At Home
Medical alert systems offer GPS enabled and at-home options so that you or your loved one can stay safe anywhere.

Don't Fall!
I'm Falling but, I'm getting up!

Portable equipment like the classic guardian by Medical Guardian even have backup batteries that can last up to 32 hours.

6. Discreet

Having an alert system doesn't have to draw attention everywhere you go. Medical alert equipment includes portable alert buttons that users can wear discreetly on their belt, wrist or neck.

7. Saves Costs on Ambulance

A single ambulance ride can cost around a thousand dollars, regardless of whether the ambulance was needed or not. You can avoid this costly hassle when using an alert device as it will connect the wearer to a trained professional who can either send an ambulance, a family member or a neighbor.

8. Easy to Use

One of the best things about medical alert devices is their simplicity. Getting help simply requires the push of a button, meaning all users can easily use the system even if it is dark or if they are visually impaired. Operators on standby

Don't Fall!
I'm Falling but, I'm getting up!

can contact medical professionals
immediately in the event of a health
emergency.

9. Works without Power
Medical alert equipment runs on long-
lasting batteries. Even in a blackout,
storm, or earthquake, medical alert
systems provide reliable assistance.

10. Reliable
At the end of the day, it comes down to
keeping loved ones safe. Many medical
alert devices such as ADT Health also
come equipped with important features
like fall detection to ensure reliable help
when you need it the most. With 24/7
monitoring capabilities, getting help is as
simple as pushing a button.

https://www.thetop10sites.com/medical-
alerts/blog/benefits-of-medical-alert-
systems.html
Check out our full list for the
best Medical Alerts 2019

In Home Medical Alert Features and
Benefits

Don't Fall!
I'm Falling but, I'm getting up!

You Need to know
1.Medical Guardian
What is a medical Guardian?
Medical Guardian is a provider of personal medical alert systems, alert monitoring and dispatch of emergency services. Whether you spend most of your time at home or are fully active, Medical Guardian has a medical alert system to suit your lifestyle.

2. Medical Alert
Easy to use, portable systems. 24/7 monitoring & flexible pricing
MedicAlert® Medical IDs
Nothing secures your <u>protection</u> more than the original medical ID from MedicAlert Foundation. More than just a MedicAlert ID, your bracelet or necklace are globally recognized and provide a full suite of emergency response services with membership.

3.Philips Lifeline
Philips Lifeline is an easy-to-use medical alert system that lets you summon help any time of the day or night – even if you can't speak. All you have to do is press your medical alert button, worn on a

Don't Fall!
I'm Falling but, I'm getting up!

wristband or pendant, and a trained Personal Response Associate will ensure you get help fast.

That's why Philips Lifeline provides the #1 Medical Alert System to offer you something else: peace of mind. Dependability is key to peace of mind. That's why doctors, hospitals and professional caregivers trust our Medical Alert.
Customized medical alert plans

In Home Medical Alert Features and Benefits

4. Life Station For the most affordable protection in and around your home, Life Station's In Home Medical Alert gives you the independence and peace of mind that comes with the leading medical alert device in America!

To see ways to make your home life easier and safer, see our Assistive Technology Devices article.
https://www.seniorliving.org/health/fall-prevention/

Don't Fall!
I'm Falling but, I'm getting up!

Chapter 15 CDC.

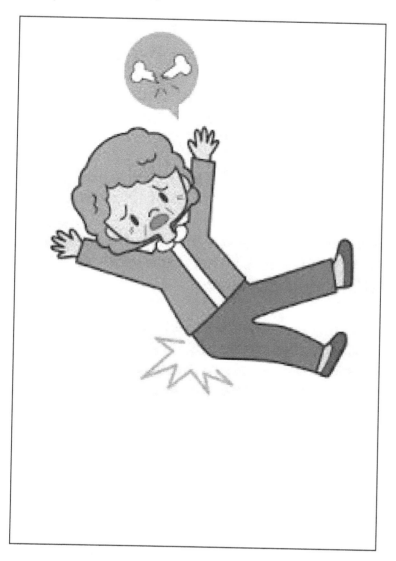

Don't Fall!
I'm Falling but, I'm getting up!

HEALTH Problem of Falls

The CDC Injury Center's Response to the Growing Public Health Problem of Falls Among Older Adults
Older adult falls are a significant cause of morbidity and mortality in the United States.

This leading cause of injury in adults aged 65 and older results in $35 billion in direct medical costs.
Objective. To project the number of older adult falls by 2030 and the associated lifetime medical cost.

A secondary objective is to review what clinicians can do to incorporate
falls screening and prevention into their practice for community-dwelling older adults.

Methods. Using the Centers
for Disease Control and Prevention's Web-based Injury Statistics Query and Reporting System and the US Census Bureau data, the number of older adults in 2030, fatal falls, and medical costs

Don't Fall!
I'm Falling but, I'm getting up!

associated with fall injuries was
projected.
 In addition, evidence-based interventions
that can be integrated into clinical
practice were reviewed. Results. The
number of older adult fatal falls is
projected to reach 100 000 per year by
2030 with an associated cost of $100
billion.

By integrating screening for falls risk into
clinical practice, reviewing and modifying
medications, and recommending vitamin
D supplementation, physicians can
reduce future falls by nearly 25%.

Conclusion. Falls in older adults will
continue to rise substantially and become
a significant cost to our health care
system if we do not begin to focus on
prevention in the clinical setting.
Falls are leading cause of injury and death
in older Americans
Healthcare providers play an important
role in falls prevention
Press Release
Embargoed Until: Thursday, September
22, 2016, 1:00 p.m. ET

Don't Fall!
I'm Falling but, I'm getting up!

Contact: Media Relations
(404) 639-3286
Every second of every day in the United States an older adult fall, making falls the number one cause of injuries and deaths from injury among older Americans.

In 2014 alone, older Americans experienced 29 million falls causing seven million injuries and costing an estimated $31 billion in annual Medicare costs, according to a new report published by the Centers for Disease Control and Prevention in this week's Morbidity and Mortality Weekly Report (MMWR).

The new numbers are being released in conjunction with the 9th Falls Prevention Awareness Day, sponsored by the National Council on Aging (NCOA). The observance addresses the growing public health issue and promotes evidence-based prevention programs and strategies to reduce the more than 27,000 fall deaths in older adults each year.

"Older adult falls are increasing and, sadly, often herald the end of independence," said CDC Director Tom

Don't Fall!
I'm Falling but, I'm getting up!

Frieden, M.D., M.P.H. "Healthcare providers can make fall prevention a routine part of care in their practice, and older adults can take steps to protect themselves."
With more than 10,000 older Americans turning 65 each day, the number of fall-related injuries and deaths is expected to surge, resulting in cost increases unless preventive measures are taken.

Don't Fall!
I'm Falling but, I'm getting up!

Chapter 16 STEADI

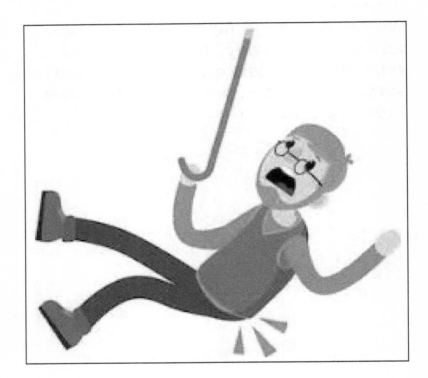

Don't Fall!
I'm Falling but, I'm getting up!

STEADI helps healthcare providers make fall prevention routine
To reduce older adult falls, CDC created the Stopping Elderly Accidents, Deaths, and Injuries (STEADI) initiative to help healthcare providers make fall prevention routine. STEADI is based on clinical guidelines and provides information and resources for patients, caregivers, and all members of the healthcare team.

STEADI includes:
Information on how to screen for falls
Online training for providers
Videos on how to conduct functional assessments Informational brochures for providers, patients and caregivers.

At CDC, we're working with healthcare providers to help keep older adults safe from falls. It all starts with three steps that healthcare providers can easily integrate into routine office visits.

At each visit, healthcare providers should:
Ask patients if they have fallen in the past year, feel unsteady, or worry about falling.

Don't Fall!
I'm Falling but, I'm getting up!

Review medications and stop, switch, or reduce the dose of medications that could increase the risk of falls.
"Falls threaten older Americans' independence and safety and generate enormous economic and personal costs that affect everyone," said Grant Baldwin, Ph.D., M.P.H., director of CDC's Division of Unintentional Injury Prevention. "Together, everyone can reduce the risk of falling and prevent fall injuries."

Reduced muscle strength, increased inactivity, more severe chronic health conditions, and increased use of prescription medications are risk factors for falls among older Americans. Fall injury rates are almost seven times higher for older adults with poor health than for those with excellent health.
https://journals.sagepub.com/doi/abs/10.1177/1559827615600137
https://www.cdc.gov/media/releases/2016/p0922-older-adult-falls.html

How older adults can reduce their risk of falling
Older adults also can take simple steps to prevent a fall:

Don't Fall!
I'm Falling but, I'm getting up!

Talk to your healthcare provider about falls and fall prevention. Tell your provider if you've had a recent fall. Although one out of four older Americans falls each year, less than half tell their doctor.
Talk to your provider or pharmacist about medications that may make you more likely to fall.

Have your eyes checked by an eye doctor once a year. Update eyeglasses as needed.
Participate in evidence-based programs (like Tai Chi) that can improve your balance and strengthen your legs.
Contact your local Council on Aging for information about what is available in your community.

Make your home safer by getting rid of fall hazards.
Recommend vitamin D supplements
For more information on the NCOA, see https://www.ncoa.org/.
For more information on CDC's STEADI initiative, see https://www.cdc.gov/steadi.

Don't Fall!
I'm Falling but, I'm getting up!

For more information about Administration on Community Living falls prevention programs, see www.aoa.acl.gov/AoA_Programs/HPW/Falls_Prevention/index.aspx.
U.S. DEPARTMENT OF HEALTH AND HUMAN SERVICES external icon

Don't Fall!
I'm Falling but, I'm getting up!

Chapter 17 Supplemental Fallers.

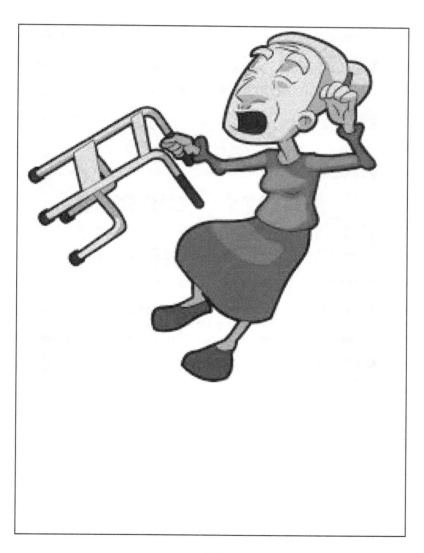

Don't Fall!
I'm Falling but, I'm getting up!

Listed here:
Famous Fallers

Everyone falls down. Falls are not only limited to people with certain income level or socioeconomic class. Falls happen to famous people as well. You'll find that falls are more common than you think.

THOSE WHO HAD RECENT FALLS
In the Arts and Entertainment
Ann B. Davis, who played Alice the housekeeper on the popular 1960s sitcom The Brady Bunch, died on Sunday in San Antonio after entering into a coma sustained by a fall in her bathtub. She was 88 years old.

On January 19th, 2013, veteran news journalist Barbara Walters, 83, missed a step and fell on a staircase at the British Ambassador's residence in Washington D.C. prior to President Obama's second inauguration. Hospitalized to treat a cut on her forehead and subsequent low-grade fever, Walters reported that she expects to be home soon.
On May 25, 2012, musician Doc Watson, 89, fell in his home. After being taken to

Don't Fall!
I'm Falling but, I'm getting up!

the hospital, it was determined he did not break any bones, but needed to undergo <u>colon</u> surgery and is in critical but stable condition.

In April 2012, Kurt Masur, the eighty-four-year-old former director of the New York Philharmonic, fell off the podium into the audience while conducting in France. He was taken to the hospital where no major injuries were found.

Actor Robert Culp, best known for his role in the hit 1960s TV show, "I Spy," died after falling in his Hollywood home on March 24th, 2010.

Dave Freeman, whose book "100 Things To Do Before You Die" inspired the recent film "The Bucket List", died after hitting his head from a fall at his home. He was 47.

Famed country singer Eddy Arnold, who's career included 28 No. 1 records, broke his hip when he fell at his Brentwood, KY home. He recently passed away while at a Nashville, TN area care facility.

Don't Fall!
I'm Falling but, I'm getting up!

Legendary UCLA <u>basketball</u> coach John Wooden fell in his condominium on Friday, February 29th, 2008, breaking his wrist and collarbone. Wooden was admitted to a local hospital and it is expected he will make a full recovery.

Beyoncé Knowles, one of the most popular singers in the world today, fell during a concert. Performing in central Florida on July 24th, 2007, Knowles tripped on her dress while trying to descend a flight of stairs. The singer fell and landed on her face, but was well enough to continue on with her routine.

Paula Abdul is known for her bubbly but benign feedback to contestants on the hit show, American Idol. On May 22, 2007, however, the gorgeous and spunky media diva fell while trying not to step on a much smaller set of toes – those of her pet Chihuahua. While "chubby little Tulip" escaped unscathed, the forty-four-year-old former cheerleader suffered bruising from her arm to her hip, a fractured toe and a broken nose.

Don't Fall!
I'm Falling but, I'm getting up!

Acclaimed author Kurt Vonnegut passed away on April 11th, 2007 due to complications from brain injuries he sustained from a fall at his Manhattan home.

Musician Ryan Adams had a fall during a concert in the UK in 2004.
Tony-winning star of the Broadway musical "Wicked" Idina Menzel fell during her performance and cracked a lower rib in January 2005.

Joe Bauman, who hit 72 home runs in 1954 playing for a minor league team in Roswell, N.M., setting a single season record for professional baseball that stood for nearly half a century, died in 2005 at a hospital in Roswell. He was 83 (see the related story).

Frank Butler OBE, 89, one of Britain's best-known sports writers, passed away in hospital on Jan 29th of 2006 following a fall at his home in Chislehurst, Kent. He was a sports editor of the News of the World for 25 years and retired 23 years ago. He covered boxing from the era of Joe Louis, was a former chairman of the

Don't Fall!
I'm Falling but, I'm getting up!

Boxing Writers Club and former steward of the British Boxing Board of Control. British jazz piano icon Mr. George Shearing was admitted to a New York City hospital after a fall in his home in March 2004.

Consuelo Velazquez, composer of the sustaining 1940s-era hit "Besame Mucho" suffered a fall at home in Mexico City in November 2004 that left her in intensive care. She recently passed away at age 88.

Kelsey Grammer, the star of the hit television comedy "Frasier" took a fall while on stage as the master of ceremonies at California Disneyland's 50th anniversary celebration in May 2005. Fortunately, the actor was not seriously hurt.

Ed McMahon, Johnny Carson's former sidekick tripped and fell in his home on March 4, 2005. McMahon, 82 suffered from a mild concussion and a gash in his head that required stitches. He was released from the Los Angeles area hospital a few days later.

Don't Fall!
I'm Falling but, I'm getting up!

Nancy Reagan, the 84-year-old widow of former US president Ronald Reagan, was briefly treated in a British hospital after she fell in her <u>hotel</u> room in London.

Robert H. Sigholtz, 84, who was general manager of Robert F. Kennedy Memorial Stadium and the D.C. Armory complex as well as athletic director at Georgetown University, died in 2005 in a hospice in Scottsdale, Ariz. He had been injured in a fall at his home in Paradise Valley, Ariz.

In Politics
Secretary of State Hillary Clinton had another fall, this time while boarding a plane. On January 12th, 2011, the former First Lady was traveling to Yemen when she tripped and fell while walking into the plane, but was unhurt.

Former First Lady and current Secretary of State Hillary Clinton fell and broke her elbow on June 17th, 2009 while walking on her way to the White House.
Supreme Court justice Sonia Sotomayor fell and broke her ankle on

Don't Fall!
I'm Falling but, I'm getting up!

June 8th, 2009, while rushing through New York's LaGuardia airport.
Former First Lady Nancy Reagan was hospitalized after home on Sunday, February 17th. She was released after a brief, 2-night stay.

Supreme Court Chief Justice John Roberts fell while at his vacation home in Port Clyde, Maine. Chief Justice Roberts was taken to the hospital as a precautionary measure and it was later determined that the fall was caused by a seizure sustained by the Chief Justice. According to sources, Roberts fell 5 to 10 feet, which caused only minor scrapes and bruises. He is expected to stay overnight in a local hospital as a precaution.

The nation's first Commissioner on Aging died after complications from a fall. William D. Bechill was one of the nation's leading experts on Social Security, long-term care and senior centers.

Mr. Bechill also played a critical role in writing the Older Americans Act, which allowed for grants supporting community

Don't Fall!
I'm Falling but, I'm getting up!

service programs, research and training
projects in the field of ageing.
Former Democratic presidential
candidate George McGovern was
hospitalized on December 2nd, 2011 after
he fell and hit his head on the
pavement while entering a library bearing
his name, where he was set to be
interviewed on C-SPAN.

In International News
Cuban President Fidel Castro tripped and
fell after leaving the stage at a graduation
ceremony in October 2004.

Mexican pop star Juan Gabriel suffered in
a fall from a stage during a performance in
Houston in 2005. Gabriel fell just minutes
into the opening set of his performance at
the <u>Toyota Center</u> and broke his wrist and
suffered a concussion.

Queen Mother suffered a slight fall and cut
her arm in her sitting room at
Sandringham in February 2002.
In Medicine

Dr. Robert Atkins, the "weight-loss guru"
that brought to us the famous "Atkins diet"

Don't Fall!
I'm Falling but, I'm getting up!

died on April 17, 2003 in New York from head injuries suffered in a fall near his office. He was 72.

In Journalism
Alistair Cooke known for his BBC series "Letter from America." suffered a fall in his Manhattan home in October 2003. Read one journalist's farewell to "the best broadcaster on four continents."

In Religion
Pope Benedict XVI underwent surgery to repair his wrist after he fell and broke it while walking in his room on July 17th, 2009.

The Rev. Harry R. Butman, a Congregational church minister for 72 years and a prolific writer about theology and the spiritual life, has passed away. He was 101.Butman died in 2005 at his home in Acton of complications from a fall.

Marj Carpenter, the ex-director of the Presbyterian News Service fell and suffered a broken hip in November 2000

Don't Fall!
I'm Falling but, I'm getting up!

while trying to enter a car outside her home in Texas.

Billy Graham, the popular evangelist who at 86 years old, suffered from two falls in 2004 that resulted in fractures. After his recuperation, he has been able to continue traveling and preaching,

FALLS   References
Bergen G, Stevens MR, Burns ER. <u>Falls and Fall Injuries Among Adults Aged ≥65 Years — United States, 2014.</u> MMWR Morb Mortal
Wkly Rep 2016; 65:993–998. DOI: http://dx.doi.org/10.15585/mmwr.mm6537a2

Stevens JA, Ballesteros MF, Mack KA, Rudd RA, DeCaro E, Adler G. Gender differences in seeking care for falls in the aged Medicare Population. Am J Prev Med 2012;43:59–62.

O'Loughlin J et al. Incidence of and risk factors for falls and injurious falls among the community-dwelling elderly. American journal of epidemiology, 1993, 137:342-54.

Don't Fall!
I'm Falling but, I'm getting up!

Alexander BH, Rivara FP, Wolf ME. The cost and frequency of hospitalization for fall–related injuries in older adults. American Journal of Public Health 1992;82(7):1020–3.

Sterling DA, O'Connor JA, Bonadies J. Geriatric falls: injury severity is high and disproportionate to mechanism. Journal of Trauma–Injury, Infection and Critical Care 2001;50(1):116–9

Centers for Disease Control and Prevention, National Center for Injury Prevention and Control. <u>Web–based Injury Statistics Query and Reporting System (WISQARS)</u> [online]. Accessed August 5, 2016.

Healthcare Cost and Utilization Project (HCUP). 2012. Agency for Healthcare Research and Quality, Rockville, MD. http://hcupnet.ahrq.govExternal. Accessed 5 August 2016.

Hayes WC, Myers ER, Morris JN, Gerhart TN, Yett HS, Lipsitz LA. Impact near the hip dominates fracture risk in elderly

Don't Fall!
I'm Falling but, I'm getting up!

nursing home residents who fall. Calcif Tissue Int 1993;52:192-198.
Parkkari J, Kannus P, Palvanen M, Natri A, Vainio J, Aho H, Vuori I, Järvinen M.

Majority of hip fractures occur as a result of a fall and impact on the greater trochanter of the femur: a prospective controlled hip fracture study with 206 consecutive patients. Calcif Tissue Int, 1999;65:183–7.

Jager TE, Weiss HB, Coben JH, Pepe PE. Traumatic brain injuries evaluated in U.S. emergency departments, 1992–1994. Academic Emergency Medicine 2000&359;7(2):134–40.
Florence CS, Bergen G, Atherly A, Burns ER, Stevens JA, Drake C. Medical Costs of

Fatal and Nonfatal Falls in Older Adults. Journal of the American Geriatrics Society, 2018 March, DOI:10.1111/jgs.15304

Vellas BJ, Wayne SJ, Romero LJ, Baumgartner RN, Garry PJ. Fear of falling and restriction of mobility in elderly fallers. Age and Ageing 1997;26:189–193.

Don't Fall!
I'm Falling but, I'm getting up!

Debra Houry, MD, MPH, <u>Curtis Florence</u>, PhD, <u>Grant Baldwin</u>, PhD, MPH, ...

First Published August 18, 2015 Research
https://doi.org/10.1177/1559827615600137

List of Sources:
<u>Aging.com</u>
<u>Centers for Disease Control and Prevention</u>

"Otago and Proven Exercises for Fall Prevention."
<u>https://www.cdc.gov/steadi/patient.html#</u>
<u>https://www.cdc.gov/steadi/patient.html#</u>

<u>https://homecareassistance.com/blog/4-long-term-consequences-of-falls-among-older-adults</u>
<u>https://medalerthelp.org/falls-in-the-elderly-statistics/</u>

<u>https://www.cdc.gov/steadi/patient.html#</u>
<u>https://www.aafp.org/afp/2010/0701/p81.html</u>

Sketches by my Grandson,

Nicholas Corsino.   Thanks Nick!

Don't Fall!
I'm Falling but, I'm getting up!

CPSIA information can be obtained
at www.ICGtesting.com
Printed in the USA
LVHW090818161019
634126LV00035B/626/P